Time and Aging
Conceptualization and Application in
Sociological and Gerontological Research

Time and Aging
Conceptualization and Application in
Sociological and Gerontological Research

Ephraim H. Mizruchi,
Barry Glassner
Thomas Pastorello
Syracuse University
Maxwell Policy Center on Aging

GENERAL HALL, INC.
Publishers
23–45 Corporal Kennedy Street
Bayside, New York 11360

TIME AND AGING
Conceptualization and Application in
Sociological and Gerontological Research

GENERAL HALL, INC.
23-45 Corporal Kennedy Street
Bayside, New York 11360

Publisher: Ravi Mehra
Editor: Susan O. Cohen
Composition: *Graphics Division,* General Hall, Inc.

LIBRARY OF CONGRESS CATALOG CARD NUMBER: 82-80240
ISBN: 0-930390-40-7
    0-930390-41-5

Manufactured in the United States of America

Contents

115306

ACKNOWLEDGEMENTS

This publication is an outcome of the activities of the Maxwell Policy Center on Aging at Syracuse University. A number of people have been directly and indirectly involved in the activities of the Center. These include Roy Price, George Zito, Jerry Jacobs, Judith Long Laws, Robert Famighetti, Beverly Klimkowski, Richard Laverdure, Anthony Kouzi, Nancy Osgood, Marilyn Nouri and Bruce Berg as well as those colleagues whose participation in the Working Conference on Time in the Social Sciences and Aging-Gerontology is reflected in their presentations and comments published here. We particularly wish to thank John Hall whose contributed paper does not appear here but whose contribution to the symposium was significant.

We gratefully acknowledge the support of the Administration on Aging through a grant to the All-University Gerontology Center; the Research Fund of Syracuse University; and the Maxwell School. Donald Kibbey and Gershon Vincow, former Vice Presidents for Research and Graduate Affairs; Alan Campbell and Guthrie Birkhead, former and current deans of the Maxwell School; Walter Beattie and Neal Bellos of the All-University Gerontology Center; and Gary Spencer, Chair of the Department of Sociology, all contributed in significant ways to the successful implementation of the working conference on which this book is based. Mary Sherman was particularly helpful in the preparation of the manuscript. Finally we thank all of the participants in the conference who provided the material for an extremely stimulating exchange.

E.H.M.
B.G.
T.P.

Syracuse, New York

INTRODUCTION

Durkheim (1965) noted that time is developed in, and affects, social life. As he put it: "It is not my time that is thus arranged; it is time in general, such as it is objectively thought of by everybody in a single civilization.... What the category of time expresses is a time common to the group, a social time, so to speak (23)."

The sociological importance and construction of time has been investigated in a variety of ways since Durkheim's pioneering discussion (Sorokin and Merton, 1937; Berger and Luckmann, 1966; Schutz and Luckmann, 1973; Roth, 1963; DeGrazia, 1962; Kolaja, 1969; Moore, 1963; Mead, 1959; Gurvitch, 1964).

This book is an attempt to extend the study of the sociology of time to a substantive area in which the importance of time cannot be overestimated — the sociology of aging. For this purpose the staff of the Maxwell Policy Center on Aging at Syracuse University invited papers from some of the leading scholars on the sociology and social philosophy of time and aging.

Jon Hendricks of the University of Kentucky is the author of *Aging in Mass Society: Myths and Realities* and *Time in the Social Sciences*. His papers on the sociology of time have appeared in a variety of publications.

Thomas Pastorello of the Syracuse University, School of Social Work, is the author of a number of papers in gerontology.

Harold L. Sheppard of the Center on Work and Aging at the American Institute for Research in Washington, D.C. has published frequently on life-span allocation of time, the economics of aging, the importance of the older worker, the retraining of older workers, and retirement.

Barry Schwartz of the University of Georgia is the author of the book, *Queuing and Waiting: Studies in the Social Organization of Access and Delay*. He has published papers concerning

1

time in social systems, the social ecology of time barriers, and time in the metropolis.

Ephraim H. Mizruchi is the former director of the Maxwell Policy Center on Aging at Syracuse University and author of *Success and Opportunity* and editor of *The Substance of Sociology.* He has published and presented papers concerning deviance, aging, sociological theory, and other topics in numerous journals and professional publications.

Eviatar Zerubavel of the department of Sociology at Columbia University has published papers in *Sociological Inquiry, American Sociological Review* and elsewhere on the social organization of time, timetables and scheduling, and calendars.

J.T. Fraser is founder and secretary of the International Society for the Study of Time. He is editor of *The Voices of Time, The Study of Time,* and *Time as Conflict.*

The authors were all invited to comment upon the others' papers. In addition, we brought together a group of scholars as discussants for the seven papers. These distinguished participants have all contributed to the literature on the sociology of aging.

Walter M. Beattie is the former director of the All-University Gerontology Center at Syracuse University and has published papers on aging in journals including *Public Welfare, The Phylon, The Gerontologist,* and *Foundation News.*

Leonard D. Cain, of Portland State University, is the author of a number of articles and book chapters in sociology and gerontology including "Life Course and Social Structure" in R.E.L. Faris, ed., *Handbook of Modern Sociology,* Chicago: Rand McNally, 1964.

Glynn Cochrane of Syracuse University is author of *Big Men and Cargo Cults, Development Anthropology, What We Can Do for Each Other,* and other books. His papers have appeared in journals including *Man, Sociologus,* and *Human Organization.*

Wallace Davis formerly of SUNY Stony Brook has published in *Journal of Cross Cultural Psychology* and the *American Journal of Sociology.*

Barry Glassner of Syracuse University is the author of *Clinical*

Sociology, Essential Interactionism and papers in *Urban Life, Urban Education, Symbolic Interaction* and elsewhere.

John R. Hall of the University of Missouri is the author of *The Ways Out: Utopian Communal Groups in an Age of Babylon* and has published papers on phenomenology, politics, and social change.

Helena Znaniecki Lopata, of Loyola University in Chicago, is the author of a number of books and articles including *Occupation: Housewife* and *Widowhood in an American City*.

Kimball P. Marshall of Washington University, St. Louis, has published papers on aging and methodology in *Sex Roles, Sociological Methods and Research* and *Sociological Quarterly*.

Victor Marshall, of the University of Toronto is the author of *Aging in Canada* and *Sociology of Aging and Dying*.

Rolf Monge of Syracuse University was Chairperson of the Department of Psychology. His publications on time, aging, and adolescence have appeared in the *Journal of Gerontology, Genetic Psychology Monographs, Developmental Psychology* and elsewhere.

The first paper, written by Jon Hendricks, sets both the intellectual tone of the book as well as establishes the framework for analyzing the debate on time as a dimension of social science theory and methodology as it bears on aging. Two perspectives on time are introduced by identifying their historical and conceptual roots in philosophy and nineteenth century social science.

One perspective represents a mechanistic temporal model. Events are unilinear and progressive. Time is an objective phenomenon existing without reference to human perception or social order. Social theorists utilizing such a model might view human history as itself linear, progressive and quantifiable. In opposition to this perspective is a relational model. Hendricks traces the development of this approach to the nineteenth century social theorist, Durkheim who questioned whether time was not contingent on culture, perception and the rhythms of social life.

Once time is considered as relational, Hendricks may then demonstrate how it can become a complex phenomenon. His discussion of time theorists, such as Sorokin Gurvitch, centers on how time might be decomposed into multiple and competing levels within both the individual and society. The dynamics of time are then explored in terms of how they apply to human affairs, that is, how people "act to create their temporal milieu." Hendricks presents a model, borrowed from the anthropologist Maltz, to illustrate the process through which the individual internalizes and reckons with four time frameworks (ecological, individual, social and ideational). Hendricks notes the importance of cultural symbols as a means to "interlock" the various diverse and uneven rates of these time dimensions within the individual. The person, Hendricks notes, almost unconsciously adjusts the time scales of his/her temporal world.

In his last section Hendricks attempts to move beyond time as relational by introducing the concept of lived time. In this section he explores the concept of memory and projection as they impact on the present. Lived time follows many paths, with memory organizing remembered events and ideas as they relate to the present focus of attention and consciousness. He argues that a sociological calendar might be a good conceptual tool to help describe the interplay among diverse temporal time tracks.

In the question period which followed the presentation of the paper, conference participants addressed their comments to the differential application of remembered past to the present as it bears on aging. One commentator noted the importance of the concept of queing when studying the social perception of the aged and dependent populations. If one's time agenda is dense a person may be valued since he is perceived as and perceives himself to be busy and important. Self worth may correlate with this perceived lack of time. Another participant noted the importance of Hendricks' analysis in terms of the encroachment of the symbol of the clock as the universal integrator. It was also observed that persons perceive themselves as functioning at differing ages depending on social context or social expectations. The question period also touched upon methodology as concerns the formulation of questions asked respondents in social science research and how the questions can pre-structure memory.

The second paper presented by Thomas Pastorello centers its discussion on the development of a "Time Paradigm" as a heuristic device which can foster the integration of aging theory, methodology and policy formulation by unconfounding time effects in life course data. Pastorello argues that his paradigm enables the social scientist to overcome the present methodological bottlenecks based as they are on the limitations of quantitative data analysis. Borrowing from Sorokin the concepts of sequence, duration, rate, rhythm, recurrence and routine and labeling them consequences, Pastorello adds what he considers antecedents: cohort, history and maturation. Antecedents and consequences are linked through the theoretical conceptualization of a socialization-allocation dialectic. A policy problem as it relates to aging could be considered as an asynchronization between socialization and role allocation. The Time Paradigm could then provide policy analysts with a way to think through the implicit temporal dimensions of the problem and develop approaches to offset the temporal disjunction.

Pastorello follows his presentation of the Time Paradigm with an analysis of five proposed approaches to asynchronization as related to work, education and leisure (retirement), using the paradigm's conceptual language. Pastorello demonstrates how a policy analyst might come to select one approach rather than others based on the paradigm. Further, it is suggested that research strategies might be selected through a similar analysis.

The discussion highlights an important consideration one might keep in mind when applying the socialization/allocation dialectic. One participant observed that the allocation of work roles is more definitive and finite than other non scarce roles, for example, leisure. Socialization was further discussed in terms of the manner in which socialization is relevant to and shaped by future expectations. The concept of socialization was challenged as a useful concept by one participant who noted that the static status role is not as helpful a concept as that of an evolving negotiated personal order without fixed temporal points.

Harold Sheppard's paper presents another approach to policy analysis. Unlike Pastorello, whose Time Paradigm provides a conceptual and theoretical framework for understanding how a problem might be defined and for selecting among policy alternatives with which to address it, Sheppard uses trend analysis as the basis for policy decision making. His interpretation of trends related to aging and work, touch upon the same debate as Pastorello outlined, that is: "Has the concept of proper age for proper social function been increasingly abandoned in our thinking and planning?" In more technical terms; has the linear, cultural pattern of socialization, work and leisure (retirement) been broken up into a cyclical pattern of recurrence of the three activities in people's lives?

Although Sheppard views the latter trend, the freedom to reverse the three variables rather than work for retirement as a progressive goal, as increasingly preferred, he is aware that there may be limits to such a pattern. Nonetheless, Sheppard notes there is hope that the increasing preference for cyclical work/non-work patterns may result in people remaining in the work force longer on a part time basis and thereby reducing the burden increased longevity imposes on the young.

In terms of policy recommendations, Sheppard interprets work/non-work and longevity trends as indicating that people will need periodic retraining (socialization) over a life-time.

The discussion which follows Sheppard's paper centers on other trend analysis studies as they bear on work and aging. One commentator observed that other nations have attempted to design and implement innovative work/non-work policies. Also, the issue of retirement itself and the comtemporary debate regarding mandatory retirement was discussed. Another concern noted was the importance of distinguishing between definitions of age as chronological number or as reflective of a stage in a cyclical pattern.

In chapter IV Barry Schwartz selects the example of access and delay in medical services to explore two contentions: 1) that time as well as money can be used as a rationing device, and 2) that the consumption of services is contingent upon macro-ecological factors as well as time and money costs and social distance factors. Schwartz used NORC survey data selecting appropriate variables to reflect income, waiting time, etc.

Schwartz develops the argument that although money can substitute for time, it does not hold that money is the sole determinant of waiting time. Blacks of all incomes wait longer than whites of comparable income. However, Schwartz does not assume that institutionalized racism or organizational factors are causal but rather looks to residential segregation; that is the spacial distribution of consumers and providers of services as such special distribution effects temporal distribution.

Schwartz contends that social life can be reflected in three types of social distance; vertical (relationships based on class and income), horizontal (relationships between ethnic groups and race) and spatial distance. He adds to the three a temporal dimension. All four, he believes, are integrated in society and movement on one effects all others. Schwartz holds that services, medical and other forms of consumption, reflect macroscopic social organization; an organization with a temporal dimension.

The questions which follow challenge Schwartz to justify that lost time is perceived as a cost. It is noted that "wasting time" may be valuable to some people. The symbolic meaning of time to various persons notwithstanding, Schwartz holds that an "impatience index" can be viewed as a measure of time cost. Further, he notes that his paper attempts to clarify that not all people are free to substitute money for time if and when they might like. His focus remains on the ecological factors which he believes are salient even when other forms of social distance are considered.

In Chapter V, Ephraim H. Mizruchi introduces two concepts he believes helpful to an understanding of social structure and aging: the distinction between and importance of surplus and superfluous populations as they bear on social organization, and the process of abeyance. Both surplus and superfluous populations represent persons incapable of being absorbed into the social structure who may become a potential threat to the existing social order by virtue of the temporal disjunction between such populations and available positions in the social order. The difference between the two, Mizruchi states, is that while surplus populations can be expected to be integrated into the social structure at some future point, superfluous populations have neither a present nor a future place in the social structure.

The process which enhances or inhibits absorption of surplus populations is abeyance. "Abeyance", Mizruchi writes, "is a holding process." It is an attempt to deal with large masses of people by transforming them into objects. It operates as a method of social control on the macro, micro and mediating levels of society.

In order to examine abeyance, Mizruchi utilizes the example of the Beguines, a religious order of women which operated in the Middle Ages as a holding structure for single women. The social structural dynamics of this abeyance structure are explored followed by contemporary examples.

Mizruchi also briefly lists the factors which are associated with the rate of absorption into the social structure of a population held in abeyance. In keeping with the focus on time all have a temporal component.

Although abeyance structures operate on the organizational level, Mizruchi notes that even within organizations there are abeyance structures, e.g., transitional status.

Mizruchi accounts for individual participation in the abeyance process, noting that the process can succeed only so far as individuals are socialized for abeyance. The Deferred Gratification Pattern formulated by Schneider and Lysgaard is a helpful heuristic device in this regard. When asynchronization in the social structure occurs such an internalized pattern assists the individual in coping with a holding process.

Further, Mizruchi argues, individuals may consciously act to cushion the impact of such asynchronization. However, Mizruchi further notes that such conscious choices, albeit structurally reinforced, can lead to further asynchronization.

In concluding, Mizruchi addresses policy considerations, noting that the social structures designed to absorb the elderly are terminal rather than abeyance structures. Such structures reflect a limited definition of status vacancies available for the elderly in society. Mizruchi challenges policy makers to direct their efforts to the transformation of terminal structures for the elderly into abeyance structures in anticipation of the reintegration of the elderly into productive status vacancies.

The discussion following Mizruchi's presentation initially focused on the historical pattern of integration of the elderly into kinship networks or social structures. It then moved to a discussion of contemporary examples of abeyance structures. Discussion also addressed the contemporary shift from cohort rites of passage to legal definitions of status transition. i.e. drinking age, etc.

Eviatar Zerubavel takes up the themes and concerns introduced by Jon Hendricks in Chapter I, that is, the evolution in western civilization of the conceptualization of time as it bears on social order. Zerubavel begins his analysis by disassembling the concept of temporal regularity, the principle underlying the schedule, into sequence, duration, timing and tempo or rate. The temporal order, he observes, like other "social facts" may go unnoticed until resisted. Each of its four dimensions is analyzed and examples given from everyday life.

The second section of his paper proceeds to a consideration of the nature of the constraints such a sociotemporal order implies. Returning to his introductory comments, Zerubavel points out the variance between the sociotemporal order and the biotemporal order or even technical rationales. He provides examples, such as the conflict between the sociotemporal order of work conventions and the biotemporal circadian rhythms.

The concept of the schedule is employed to highlight the multiple inroads of sociotemporal conventions and patterning in individual lives. Zerubavel maintains that a complex civilization based on a high degree of differentiation cannot function without such social constraints which serve an integrative function. Such a sociotemporal patterning may both prevent cognitive anomie and provide normative proscription which may serve to simplify personal decision making. In concluding, Zerubavel emphasizes that temporal regularity is a social fact which in part generates the schedules under which we live and give a characteristic structure to modern social life.

The discussion which follows considers the question whether sociotemporal organization can be utilized to further freedom as well as for purposes of social control. In a long response one participant provides examples of how schedules may be used in pursuit of personal interests. Examples are given to affirm the position that temporal patterning can be used for coordination as well as control or self interest. Zerubavel agrees noting that in the presented paper he had elected to focus on control aspects.

In the concluding paper, J.T. Fraser delineates a theory of time as conflict which "sees the basic matrix of the world as an open-ended heirarchy of integrative levels --(umwelts)-- each with its particular temporality, causation, language and unresolved conflicts". Fraser borrows from natural philosophy and presents a model of evolving integrative levels from the most simple massless particles -- atemporal, no past, present or future -- to the most complex integrative level capable of being envisioned -- the sociotemporal. Evolution is seen as resulting from instability generated by unresolved conflicts within each level, although, Fraser notes, an "umwelt" can only be sustained and indeed is defined by its conflicts.

Between integrative levels remain a class of phenomena decribed as interfaces or intermediate levels. Fraser posits that the position of man in our epic is an interface between the nootemporal (focus on mind, individual) and the sociotemporal (focus on the collective/society). Fraser outlines how each of the integrative levels results from a natural selection process and maintains a language with which to comprehend lower integrative levels. The sociotemporal integrative level which Fraser envisions will in its turn subsume all lower levels including that of individual mind. However, at present, the sociotemporal may operate with a logic and language incapable of being grasped by the individual mind. Indeed, Fraser believes, conflicts presently perceived as irresolvable by the individual mind may in the future be viewed by a collective consciousness as false conflicts or unanswerable within the logic and language of the nootemporal. Fraser contends that the tension between individual and society defines the present as metastable and will be transitory. Following his logic, Fraser states that the future will either progress to the anticipated sociotemporal level or regress to lower temporal stages.

The individual mind, Fraser argues, is increasingly unable to function rapidly enough in an environment made increasingly complex by the actions of collective individual minds. Hence the individual mind may no longer be the unit of consciousness but merely a part of a larger consciousness. The alternative is to simplify the social world by breaking it down into smaller units. Examples are given, and the challenge to social science research posed. In response to present instability, Fraser envisions a revolt not against persons or externals but a revolt against the unresolved conflicts of the mind.

Chapter **1** TIME AND SOCIAL
SCIENCE: HISTORY AND
POTENTIAL

Jon Hendricks, Ph. D.
Department of Sociology
University of Kentucky

While time and temporality are central to much of the sociological enterprise, our conceptualizations have thus far remained largely underdeveloped. Despite occasional contentions that time is as much a part of our socially constructed reality as any other component of our worldview, only in isolated instances have we taken a closer look at what at first glance appears to be both inpenetrable and manifestly obvious.

After all, common sense and much of science alike would have us believe that neither time's cadence nor its direction is open to question. Consequently, the relevance of time in social science has been ambiguously defined, cast mostly in an implicit role, presumably known and understood without further attention required. Unfortunately, the model of time adopted by social science disciplines from classical mechanics and Newton's seminal contributions has itself been superseded.

Even Einstein, whose formulation of relativity theory will stand as a milestone in the mapping of time's course, grew discontented with completely physical, pre-emptive conceptions of time. In fact, according to Whitrow, he called into question the very underpinnings upon which our temporal monism has been founded. As Whitrow points out, despite time's naturalistic features, it is also a subjective social phenomenon, which he claims ultimately leads Einstein to conclude that in certain respects time is a component of our consciousness lacking any so-called physical objectivity (Whitrow, 1972:166).

12

In order to suggest an alternative to the dominant physical character accorded time in the social sciences, it is necessary to first become acquainted with the genesis and main themes of two alternative views. Having gained some understanding of their constitution our attention will then be directed to an exploration of the pragmatic ramifications of these as they are utilized in the creation of temporal orientations in the course of everyday life.

TWO VIEWS OF TIME

Primacy of Physical Time

Somewhat surprisingly, the most pervasive model of time in sociology in particular is one which contends time is indeed an objective phenomenon, totally equatable with its measure. In short, it is a position taken from the proposition that time is an ontological entity existing independently of our perception of it, flowing continuously onward--each moment the same as that which preceded it. There is of course an alternative view, one in which time is cast as a social construct, derived from determinate intentional frames of reference. Here, time is not seen as an interval scale but rather it runs discontinuously, colored by a plurality of contextual factors. While both of these views have a long tradition, it is the contention of this paper that the first is incapable of handling certain essential features of our temporal awareness. In fact, to go further, it is incumbent upon all social scientists to heed the admonishment Sorokin and Merton (1937) offered over forty years ago. "It is a gratuitous assumption that astronomical or even calendrical time systems are best fitted for designating and measuring simultaneity, sequence, and duration of social phenomena."

The image of temporality which began by linking it to motion and ultimately came to conceive of time as an absolute categorical reality can be traced back through Newton to Aristotle. For Aristotle (1961, iv. 11. 220a, 26-28), time is seen as dependent on a realization of motion, since motion is inherent in the universe so too is time--thus it is objectively real. With the rise of the modern scientific method following the Copernican revolution, modifications were made in the cosmological assumptions underlying ideas about time.

The heritage of these Newtonian reformulations is a focus on the exogenous character of time, arising from ongoing physical processes not related to the perceiving subject. In essence, time is presumed to be ontologically prior to consciousness of it, characterized by Eddington (1958) as seemingly following its own arrow. Over the course of the eighteenth and nineteenth centuries it is but a short step from the quantifiable time of the physical world to an application of these same principles to analysis of the temporal nature of the social world. History and the shaping of change in individual as well as societal level phenomena were thought of as following an analogous arrow. Allowing for alterations in underlying teleological presuppositions, most of the early social theorists who sought to explicate the forces of social change adopted the casual framework inherent in the mechanistic temporal model which was central to Newtonian science. From Turgot and Condorcet to Comte, Spencer, even Marx, nearly all sociologists and their brethren placed their bets on an incremental accumulation of unilinear time--from past to present to a future yet to come (Gilb, 1966).

The overriding image of the temporal environment fostered by the new scientific worldview were being buttressed at the same time by the emerging technological rationality of industrialism. Gradually our notions of time came to be completely secularized, granted a commodity-like status and accordingly not receptive of further inquiry (Woodcock, 1944; Rezsohazy, 1972). It was not merely the hardware of the techniques which prompted this ascendency but the entire conceptual underpinning which was responsible for altering humanity's worldview (Johnson, 1972; Heise, Lenski and Wardwell, 1976). So pervasive was the transformation that Mumford suggests clocks, those prophetic exemplars of the embryonic industrial era, not machines *per se*, provided the symbolic integration necessary for the restructuring of everyone's life. As the dominance of an independent isochronal clock time grew exponentially, following the introduction of mechanical escapements in the mid-fourteenth century, it became the primary referential standard to which all other periodizations of life were subjected. As the prevalence of clocktime spread, the whole notion of temporality came to be disassociated not only from its religious origins but from the reality of human events, indeed quite the reverse quickly became the case; such time as was denoted by timekeeping devices imposed its own regimented order on the world (Berger, 1977; Mumford, 1934; see also Durkheim, 1915).

RELATIONAL TIME

Challenges to the ontological status of time inherent in Newtonian mechanics emerged from two quarters. First, from the realm of physics, relativity theory unsettled the entire conceptual framework. Einstein (1964) himself maintained that the notion of absolute time derived from the spatial coordinates implied in classical physics was arbitrary at best. Utilizing his own critical appraisal of the model, based in part on his reading of Hume and Mach, Einstein concluded that the two basic premises of classic mechanics, though each was based on experience, were ultimately incompatible. Accordingly, he departed from the purely mechanical model of Newton by locating the basic data of physics in energy rather than matter. In its place Einstein theorized that the number of times must correspond to the number of frames of reference, differing according to diverse levels of analysis and the perspective of the observer. As a consequence, he realized that in physics and other natural sciences the multifaceted nature of time entails a plurality of measures each dependent on the events in question and the vantage point from which they are viewed.

In terms of our own discipline, a second stream of thought, running in opposition to time as an absolute, flows from Augustine to Bergson to Husserl thence spreads out as a counter current in sociology through the work of Mannheim, Sorokin, Gurvitch and others (Hendricks and Hendricks, 1976). As in relativity theory, this orientation considers time as an epiphenomenal multifaceted variable based on subjective perception; strict quantification thereby assuming a secondary role in its constitution. Just as Einstein held that the measure of time corresponds to the number of frames of reference, those social scientists who think of time as a constitutive element of experience maintain a complex relational concept of time better suited to the flux of daily life. The criticism often heard is that objective clock time is a coercive factor in the study of humanity, and, since it is exogenous, hardly the most relevant view of time for sociologists in their analysis of on-going activities. Sorokin summarized the objections succinctly when he insisted:

> . . .that the social sciences cannot be adequately served by any of the physio-mathematical, biological, and psychological times and need an adequate conception of sociocultural time as one of their main referential principles (1964, 158).

In contrast to the Aristotelian equation of time and motion as inherent properties of the universe, Augustine asserted back in the fifth century that time demands a mind apart from the universe if it is to be recognized. Putting aside the theological baggage and his ontological assumptions about the soul, Augustine's heritage is that the constitutive nature of temporality is a matter of activity and of perception--time is that which in passing characterizes consciousness. Hence even if motion were to cease, the memory of it, and thus of time, would continue to exist in the present. In fact, both past and future must exist in the present if they are *to be* at all. For Augustine, anticipating the Kantian twist on the intuiting subject, it is the soul--defined variously but for our purposes here, as a God-fearing self-conscious actor will not be unjust--which permits past and future to be. Past events do not in themselves exist, only the image of them in the memory of the soul. Similarly, when we predict the future it is not tomorrow we see but the foreshadowings of it in the present of the soul. Outside the soul only the present can exist, but in consciousness there is memory, attention, anticipation. In the soul--in the consciousness of the actor--there is a present memory of past events, a present attention to present events, and a present anticipation of future events (1953: xi, 20, 26).

Reiterating the Augustian theme, as modified however by Kant, Bergson also staked the reality of time in inner experience. He disagreed with the temporal homogeneity asserted in the Kantian view of succession, maintaining instead that the real time of duration, or lived experience, is heterogeneous and indivisible. Paradoxically, he felt that despite the qualitative character of lived experience, time itself could be broken into instants and, through the intermediary of motion, quantified (1965). Similarly, it is the consciousness of the intending actor which is key to temporality as conceived by Husserl, and by Merleau-Ponty as well, though both reject motion as the foundation. In Husserl's case, time arises with the constancy and endurance of the objects of consciousness. Thus memory, as the avenue by which consciousness compares the results of its constitutive activity, is the source of time (Husserl, 1966). Merleau-Ponty, on the other hand, denies the possibility of pure inner experience by contending that the issues of subjectivity-objectivity, internality-externality are inseparable. Yet, obviously the world exists prior to our being in it, therefore experience may describe but cannot constitute the passage of time. Rather, it stems from the actor's relation to events which, by necessity, provides a finite perspective at best, one incapable of grasping the whole. Objects exist in the world's present, but time and succession--past and future--occur only with the appearance of a self-consciously perceiving subject (1962).

TIME IN SOCIOLOGY

While few sociologists have directed prolonged attention to the subject of time, those who have investigated its nature have drawn primarily on the foregoing ideas in formulating their own interpretations of time in the social world. Although his predecessors certainly were aware of time as a socially constructed variable, Durkheim represents one of the first major figures in our discipline to explicitly address himself to the constitution of social time. As far as he is concerned, time without a process by which it can be identified is inconceivable, therefore it can be neither *a priori* nor empirical in the traditional sense. Even private experience is not sufficient since in itself it is systematized and ordered by the cultural context. As far as Durkheim is concerned, our temporal sense is a cultural artifact, flowing out of the collective memory, with a coercive influence on an individual's personal experiencing of time. In every instance he saw the function of time, and the symbolic notation through which it is maintained, as pragmatic; determined by the ebb and flow of the culture as exemplified in the periodic recurrence of rites, festivals, public ceremonies, and so on (Durkheim, 1915). In extending Durkheim's perspective, two of his disciples, Hubert and Mauss, point out that the temporal environment promulgated by particular cultures is hardly homogeneous, infinitely divisible or strictly linear--the very principles of Newtonian time. Simply stated, "there is always something else besides the quantitative considerations of more or less." The purpose of calendars, and by implication all socially relevant forms of time-keeping, is to punctuate, not measure, the rhythms of social life. Consequently, the durations between temporal landmarks are usually variable, rarely ever equivalent units. Because they are of such significance, the critical dates specified by the calendar disrupt the continuity of time's passage. Its cadence is uneven and changeable, yet the rhythms established by these socially significant demarcations are ascendent over others. In fact, it is these periodizations which are the *real* units of our time reckoning and are thus impenetrable beyond the intervals established (Hubert and Mauss, 1909). Halbwachs (1925) also relied on Durkheim for his theoretical foundation, referring to the social frameworks established by cultures as the key to memory, reflecting not merely psychological attributes, but a collective process furnishing the temporal guideposts essential to all recollection (see Sorokin,

1964 for a discussion).

Mannheim, in rejecting the objective time of classical physics, sought an alternative based on the experiencing of common influences which promote an identifiable mentality. Instead of quantitative temporal units, Mannheim defined generations as denoting episodic time flow insofar as each shares a consciousness of decisive life-events forever after coloring its members' worldview. Like Dilthey, Mannheim (1952) emphasized that contemporaneity in itself does not suffice to make a generation, cognizance of historical consciousness--a group identity forged in and by "fresh contact," or reinterpretation of existing phenomena--is required. Consequently, the "epochal" character of historical time as a macro-level phenomenon is marked by a changing *Zeitgeist*, rather than a mere passing of the years.

In his criticism of unilinear quantitative time, Sorokin treads the same path taken by Durkheim and Mannheim. Unfortunately he follows too closely, for despite his indictment of all underlying linear frameworks, Sorokin postulates an unswerving temporal succession from past to present and on to future developments (Gilb, 1966). While in Sorokin's model, social events do provide the points of reference, like Durkheim or Mannheim he allows for no variation in the on-going temporal rhythm of the collectivity. He does recognize that quantitative models cannot account for the diverse qualitative properties attributed to changes in distinctive time periods, nor can they explain the various time expressions of localized groups as they reflect the social activities of the aggregate and the interaction of their members. Even when natural or environmental factors might be employed to establish time frames, their adoption as benchmarks is dependent on their significance and utility for the group. In fact, without referential note being taken, stretches of what others might consider time will not be reckoned with or perceived according to Sorokin. In other words, only those moments which are imbued with some importance by the group are recognized--the others quickly fade away into nothingness. It is the notation of critical dates which provides temporal demarcations and interrupts the continuity postulated in Newtonian time. This process, which Sorokin labels "social time," is what gives the calendrical reference its significance--as conventional or symbolic integration of these socially important guideposts to temporal events (Sorokin and Merton, 1937; Sorokin, 1964).

For analytic purposes, Sorokin adopts the medieval system which divides the pulsation of social time into three interrelated planes: *aeternitas, aevum* and *tempus.* Leaning rather heavily on the postulates of neo-Kantian idealism, Sorokin contends that we categorically create the world of our experience through our own activity. To begin with, there is the *aeternitas* or ideational level of time, the realm of pure timeless meaning, which is eternal and unchanging, without "before " or "after", having no sequence. It is the world of non-temporal *Being,* wherein resides social-cultural values which cannot be fixed or dated. Next, the *aevum* or idealist plane of time is, as Sorokin claims, the "co-participant" of the first level. It is the historical manifestation which can be thought of as a temporal approximation of the absolute categories, changing in the particular but not in their essentiality. Generalizations based on observation, such as the propositions of science and logic, are examples of the *aevum.* They are illustrative of eternal verities, yet their realization can be dated. Finally, the sensate phenomena of life, those fleeting, ephemeral events which constitute the substance of experience exist on the *tempus* plane. Time proceeds space, depending on whether the events in question occur within the fabric of atomic, cellular, physiological or any other of the diverse social levels. Since each event is relative to its own level and functioning, specification of temporal passage is contingent on criteria which have little to do with chronology as measured by the clock. It is on this last level that most conceptions of time are formulated, although to adequately locate time, all three levels are necessary in Sorokin's view. Otherwise, temporal events are relegated to either the world of unchanging *Being* or to the sensory world, subject to the influence of every passing condition. In practical terms it is the *tempus* which lies within the focus of sociology, for through its explication the higher levels will eventually become known. To make sense of time, duration and change in the *tempus*, we must rely on pluralistic quantitative and qualitative measures since there are no universal standards, and depend on those which provide the most inclusive referential system (Sorokin, 1964).

In order to suggest an alternative to the dominant physical character accorded time in the social sciences, it is necessary to first become acquainted with the genesis and main themes of two alternative views. Having gained some understanding of their constitution our attention will then be directed to an exploration of the pragmatic ramifications of these as they are utilized in the creation of temporal orientations in the course of everyday life.

Gurvitch (1964), like Sorokin, takes social time, defined as culturally constructed multidimensional phenomena, as his point of departure. In addition, he is one of several who offer a dialectical critique of a world wherein the products of our creation are given a *real*, concrete status, divorced from our own making; granted facticity as though they had an existence apart from our intentions. Time, then, is also objectivated, cast as something whose reality is not within our control but which in its turn makes us--in short, a process of reification. From this vantage point Gurvitch presents his theory of social time as a reconstruction of temporality treated as a putative component of the lifeworld. The key element in his analysis is what he terms the *depth levels*, a vehicle for probing beyond the readily apparent surface of social reality. Attention then can be addressed to either a single level to determine, in our case with time, how events are constituted or alternatively, an attempt can be made to reveal the interrelatedness between levels as in the concatenation of the distinctive times operating on each level.

In brief, the levels Gurvitch delineates are:

(1) The *ecological surface* where geographical, environmental and climatic factors exert primacy as an arena within which all human affairs must unfold;

(2) *Organizational level* or institutionalized arrangements with their pre-existing and fixed rules constraining behavior. Though providing a less rigid backdrop than ecological factors, organizational control acts as a check against

spontaneous activity. Nonetheless, there exists a dialectical relationship between the hierarchically established criteria of the institutionalized order and the invigorating flux of daily life;

(3) *Models, rules,* and *signals* are contained in the next level wherein the conventions of particular situationally-determined norms provide consistent standards of behavior. Again, Gurvitch asserts a reciprocal interpenetration between recognized rules of conduct and on-going unstructured activity;

(4) *Social roles* follow and prescribe in still more flexible fashion the actual enactment of behavior;

(5) *Collective attitudes* are the "inponderables of the social atmosphere", or the collective consciousness as Durkheim would say, which provide the open parameters for selection among alternatives;

(6) *Symbols, ideas, collective values and cultural products* come together on the next level yet are interdependent with all the others. They serve as adumbrated mediators for the expression of the values inherent in a culture as seen from individualized perspectives;

(7) *Collective mentality* is the most difficult substratum to reach, for it is the realm "of the total psychic phenomena" (Gurvitch, 1964).

Each of these levels, delaminated for analysis but inseparably conjoined in reality, is assumed by Gurvitch to move in its own time with each interpenetrating the others and contributing to the enveloping temporal ecology. In order to avoid clashes between the varying rhythms characteristic of each level and other elements present in societal settings, a unifying hierarchy of *social time* is clearly a necessity.

Without pausing to provide a detailed overview of the durations, rhythms and orientations of the times operative on each of the depth levels, it is possible to characterize the eight kinds of time which are representative of each and which constitute the various manifestations of social time. In Gurvitch's view, these times not only exist in and on the levels themselves, but also represent time found in various macro-and micro-social aggregates. *Enduring time* is the most uninterrupted form of social time. As a projection of the past into the present and ultimately into the future, it is seemingly slowed down though perhaps it is the most easily quantified. Typically, this is the time of the ecological level. *Deceptive time* is discontinuous, hence likely to surprise, continually breaking with previous patterns. As a feature of the organizational level, it is filled with paradoxical decompositions as the institutional arrangements themselves undergo change. *Erratic time* is irregular and uncertain,· based on contingencies arising from the levels of social roles and collective attitudes. In all cases the present is utilized as a guide to the past as well as the future in a pragmatic and purposive sense. *Cyclical time* represents a confluence of past, present, and future into a single ubiquitous moment. Since it is qualitative, cyclical time is found primarily in those groups and societies still governed to some degree by magical or religious beliefs. *Retarded time* is characteristic of the social symbols and closely knit groups, it is outmoded as it is realized. As Gurvitch notes, the moments of retarded time are "jaded as soon as they are expressed" because their unfolding has been awaited so long. *Alternating time* belongs to the level of signs, rules or models as well as collective conduct which exhibits some regularity. It fluctuates between delay and advance as past, present and future compete with one another, promoting discontinuity over continuity without attention given to qualitative factors. Because it is intimately tied to economic organizations, alternating time first appeared with the advent of capitalism. *Time in advance of itself* is pushing forward in a dynamic integration of future into present. It is a time of aspirations, of protensive ideals or innovations. Generally, time in advance of itself is the time of the proletarian classes. *Explosive time* is also characterized by an emphasis on futurity but, unlike advancing time, appears most startlingly during revolutionary change; accordingly it is unstable and discontinuous. Since past and present are subverted in the interest of future concerns, explosive time is often associated with centralized collectivities, though in capitalist states it may appear as a pretension leading ultimately to instability.

Despite the ambiguity of Gurvitch's temporal pluralism, it definitely accentuates the concept of relativity sought by

Durkheim, Sorokin and his other forebears. Considerable work remains before any defensible conclusions can be reached regarding the validity, or the usefulness, of his or any of the other models claiming to capture the essence of time as a socially constructed fact of life. What has been missing thus far, at least in the sociological literature, is an attempt to demonstrate the applicability of such dynamic conceptions to the affairs of humankind. It is to a preliminary exploration of just this task that we now turn.

TIME AS EXPERIENCE

The groundwork necessary for a dynamic conception of the multiplicity of temporal coordinates has been set. Since Einstein, Bohr and others originally propounded their theories, physical scientists have come to openly acknowledge the plurality of times and the part played by the involvement of the scientists in their observation. While they do not yet have command of the requisite tools for identifying them, physicists have concluded that in the physical world times other than that which has been conceived in a unidirectional absolute form exist (Whitrow, 1961). The difficulty of constructing adequate theories of time in the social realm is equally complex. The possibility that there are numerous actively constructed temporal dimensions in the experiential world ought to be explored further before the use of the convenient mechanical model completely overshadows the role of the actor in the creation of his or her temporal milieu.

TEMPORAL STRUCTURING
IN SOCIAL SYSTEMS

To appreciate the constitutive quality of time it is essential to pause for a moment to examine the literature of anthropology as it relates to the structure of time. In doing so, it becomes readily apparent that in their analyses of non-Western cultures, social anthropologists have long recognized the relativistic nature of temporal reckoning (Bock, 1966). Furthermore, it is also generally accepted that not only does each social reality exude its own time but each type of social institution or cultural pattern within the larger social order may incorporate a particular temporal framework in its very structure (Braudel, 1972; Gluckman, 1968). While it is certainly true that many non-industrial or third world societies demonstrate no great concern about what industrial societies deem accurate or even consistent time reckoning, this, in itself, provides significant clues as to the importance of various forms of social activities and significant values (Maxwell, 1971; Heirich, 1964; Evans-Pritchard, 1940). Regardless of the fact that hunting-gathering, agrarian, and industrial societies have representative temporal frameworks, it is possible to present a summary schematic depicting the dimensions of time reckoning in non-industrial groups. Such an overview should help clarify the integration of diverse temporal orderings in the modern world as well. Finally, we shall turn to an elaboration of time perspectives as they may interrelate within the realm of individual consciousness.

Rather than review the numerous studies of time-reckoning found in the anthropological archives, a most insightful schema developed by Maltz (1968), should prove invaluable for analyzing the systemic relationship and integration of temporal levels. While Maltz's model refers to so-called primitive peoples, the applicability of its conceptual distinctions for the contemporary scene is undiminished. As is evident from the summaries of the principal approaches used to characterize time in the social sciences, and as Maltz states in his own survey of theoretical articles in anthropology, three essential problems must be addressed before it is possible to assess the nature of temporal ordering. First, how do individualized psychological components of time-reckoning relate to the social? Whether one sides with Durkheim, and assumes that despite appearances time is always social, or with Husserl, who contends that subjectivity is the origin of time, it should be obvious that these two levels interact. As Sorokin would ask, "How does socio-cultural temporality fit with personal time experience?" Second, since all social aggregates apparently have diverse temporal systems for various cultural patterns and institutions, how are these ordered and coordinated? In part this was exactly Gurvitch's concern in his attempt to formulate a depth and dialectical model. Finally, what is the fundamental nature of the particular time scales in use? That is, how are the intervals, units of measure or periodicities established in each sphere?

Without belaboring the steps taken by Maltz in his analytic synopsis of pre-industrial temporal frameworks, let us consider Figure 1 as a possibly useful way to represent how experiential time may actually be composed.

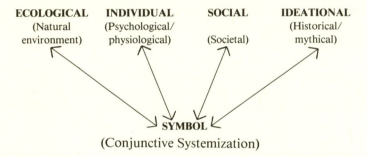

ECOLOGICAL   INDIVIDUAL   SOCIAL   IDEATIONAL
(Natural   (Psychological/   (Historical/
environment)   physiological)   (Societal)   mythical)

SYMBOL
(Conjunctive Systemization)

Figure 1. Dialectical Facets of Time as Experience (adapted from Maltz, 1968).

The descriptive labels across the top refer to the different temporal modes derived from experience. From Durkheim and Merleau-Ponty to Gurvitch, Sorokin and the ethnographic anthropologists, most observers agree environmental factors are one of the most significant contributors in organizing experience. At the outset, concrete experiential factors impose a temporal perspective on activities and events. In terms of what is labelled *ecological* time, Cope (1919), and Nilsson (1920) made clear in two early ethnographic accounts of time that nature provides a basic and fundamental calendar regulating human conduct. Generally speaking an initial dichotomy is all there is, time is linked to change; wet or dry, light or dark, warm or cold are seasons which serve to modulate subsistence activities and the reckoning of temporal durations as they exist in limited form. Later on, other aspects of the milieu are included; planting-harvesting cycles, time of the fish and so on, until in Gurvitch's view all environmental objects, both natural and created, serve a similar purpose. In short, the salient components of the environment which are imbued with acknowledged social value serve as a backdrop which initially differentiates time and its passing. What is specified as the *individual* dimension of time is intended as a reference to subjectively meaningful concrete events recognized by individuals in constructing their own temporal fields. Here it is the purposively attended to which is crucial in the determination of time. Whether time flows as a result of inner experience, as Bergson would have it, or is a reflection of external events as they impact upon the life and consciousness of individuals, as Merleau-Ponty, James and others claim, it is contingent on an active individual. Even without a fully developed conception of the future, pre-industrial people are certainly able to gauge their own relative position in the life-cycle and hence provide an elemental temporal structuring of their lifespace. Moving from fairly straight-forward physiological continuity to increasingly complex cognitive constitution of temporal horizons, individuals gear themselves into the world according to their own protensive temporal projections which possess an essential reality of their own.

On the *social* dimension, relevant time frames are synthetically, that is to say, normatively, determined. By definition, it is a shared time, wrought from the crucible of interpersonal interaction. However, because it is social, it exists apart from individuals themselves, realized by custom, extending beyond the lifetime and attention of any particular actor. Socially determined time is referential in that it provides the cultural configuration within which individual temporality is synchronized. An obvious example among both industrial and non-industrial groups is anytime people come together for a common purpose prescribed and sanctioned by "the rhythm of collective left" (Sorokin and Merton, 1937). In Gurvitch's scheme there is no single equivalent category, however his organizational models, social roles and so on, can likely be subsumed under the social label, then broken out again for analytic purposes. The remaining dimension, designated as *ideational* in Figure 1, refers to historical and mythical temporalities which serve to situate past, present and future in terms of traditions, significant historical events (those given meaning in the culture), even mythical occurrences which denote transitions in a group's character. Unlike the previous dimensions, the ideational is non-experiential and is only apparent when historical comparisons or cosmological questions are included as the frame of reference.

Despite their essential role in determining the forms of temporality characteristic of lived time, the unalloyed temporal dimensions do not automatically integrate themselves. Each is referenced through pervasive cultural symbols which impose a correspondent time track upon each dimension, thereby insuring an interlocking of their diverse and uneven rates. In short, each dimension is subordinated to a conjunctive indicia or check point, so that it can be intercalated with the others. From the numerous anthropoligical examples Maltz and others provide, it is evident that any natural or social event may be accorded symbolic significance and thus serve as a horologic reference point for time reckoning on all four dimensions. Both constancy and change, as well as duration, come to be experienced in terms of certain symbolic occurrences which are themselves repetitive. The systematization is carried out in terms of other phenomena also taken as reference points though these others may well be qualitatively different. Originally the symbols which serve as integrating or unifying mechanisms are purely local and ethnocentric in nature, based on subsistence or economic activities. As these events are routinized they often become festive occasions, marking the end of one period and the beginning of another with the festival itself used as a benchmark for events on each of the four dimensions. For example, the Thanksgiving holiday in the United States marks the end of the harvest, the beginning of the winter season, a historical event in our country's history as well as a number of personal changes. Because Thanksgiving has common emotional or cognitive meaning for all Americans, it may be considered, to use Durkheim's phrase, a "collective representation," consequently serving as a means of unifying all levels of temporal experience. In the broadest sense it is through the coercive power of collectively shared symbols that temporal stability is achieved and maintained.

The exact nature of the symbols in use depends not only on the parameters of social interaction between and within groups, but on the stage and type of social development as well (Tiryakian, 1977). As both become increasingly complex, localized temporal symbols are replaced by more abstract representations capable of communicating a temporal orientation which is interchangeable, cutting across social and cultural boundaries. While many of the symbols utilized by our non-industrial counterparts have been lost to us in the industrial era, the principle remains the same. We have merely substituted universally acceptable symbols, primarily the calendar and the clock, as integrating mechanisms. Unfortunately their priority has helped reify these two indicators to an extent that all other time orientations have been depreciated to the point of meaninglessness. In speaking to just this, Mumford (1934) notes, with more than a little irony, that it is not the steam engine but the clock which is the key machine of the industrial era, since it is the most typical and ubiquitous symbol of the modern age. One of the primary differences between the clock or the calendar and the conjunctive symbols employed in non-industrial cultures is that our system is stripped of the personalized meaning implicitly contained in the early symbols derived directly from experience. We are no longer attuned to the fact that any time coordinating symbol is merely an artifact of our desires to keep track and not something with a reality apart from our purposes.

As practical as a secularized temporal symbol may be in the technological sphere, or in terms of world-wide cooperation, its measurement by either clocks or calendars is not sufficient when the question turns to a consideration of the immediacy of the extended time of life. In a discussion of "objects from without" Locke noted long ago in his *Essays Concerning Human Understanding* that regardless of external measures of objects of events (Newtonian time included), these must be referred to a cognizance of "the working of our mind within us" and vice versa if either is to be perceived. As an illustration, what point would be served by marking something as having happened 1000 hours or even 41 days ago? Without additional reference or a conversion to a socially relevant benchmark, such a notational account is not particularly significant in terms of its placement in the flux of our lives or current events. Even with its placement clarified in terms of the annual meetings of our professional society, there is every likelihood that my colleagues will have a different recollection than my own since our lives have not followed identical patterns in the meantime, nor have the intervening temporal units been homogeneous (Stevens, 1975). Reflecting back or looking ahead in time, in fact our whole sense of duration and experience, is not a protensive linear process either, since both are colored by our particular temporal organization as influenced by the pace of the succession of our thoughts and activites.

Following Bergson, Sorokin and Merton, Gurvitch and all the others who have questioned the appropriateness of the application of Newtonian physics to the analysis of the personal experience of time, it seems that greater explication is long overdue. Actually, the construction of our personal integrating mechanisms is a multifaceted process, with each dimension applicable to different areas of life. In fact, it takes only a moment's reflection to realize the extent to which we all employ personalized special purpose time scales based on experience, memory and anticipated futures to organize our own temporal worlds. Clearly the possibility exists of numerous temporal dimensions within a single individual's experiential world. Yet little in the conceptual armory of sociology prepares us to deal with such an eventuality. It is an examination of the constitution of temporal frameworks in an individual's everyday world and one means for dealing with the dynamic of time that we now take up.

LIVED TIME

To a great extent we think of time as something which flows past an individual, receding away either into the past or fading to some other unrecoupable place. When asked how we measure this flowing temporal process, almost without reflection we turn to the standard clocks or calendars in order to ascertain time's rate. Ironically however, even that rate must then be referred to other comparative events or the relationship between events if it is to provide much meaning (Smart, 1967; Williams, 1951). In terms of individual awareness it is apparent that the overarching mechanistic conception glosses over the dynamic nature of temporality as lived experience. In their attempts to rectify this situation Halbwachs, Husserl and others have stressed the role memory plays in structuring temporal intentionality. Their concerns deserve further attention if for no other reason than there is nothing in the classical mechanistic view of time which accounts for an individual's extended sense of duration. In granting their contention that it is through memory that we realize a sense of lived experience and change, we also obligate ourselves to a closer exploration of the continuity between recollection, present and expected futures. How these three temporal realms interrelate with one another and to the question of reflexivity, to our "work of attention," is crucial in determining how temporal awareness is shaped.

Let me begin by reiterating what others have claimed, the act of paying attention is intrinsically intentional, hence can be examined in terms of dominant issues or themes. To illustrate, at the moment I am absorbed with the role of attention in organizing my life, consequently I reorganize my thoughts and recategorize my recent experience in terms of this significant task, shifting away from my previous project which was to sate the rumblings of my stomach. As I shift the locus of my attention from one project to another I implicitly shift the organizing schema of memory as well. Were I to reflect ahead on tasks or projects yet to be accomplished, the focal length of my anticipations would also reflect my present orientation. As Mead would phrase it, "reality exists in the present," which is to say, both past and future are hypothetical reconstructions interpreted from and bound together through the mental *NOW* (Mead, 1932; Natanson, 1953). In the case of my rumbling stomach I would probably cast ahead to the next meal time or in terms of my current concern to the likely conclusion of this paper. In either case the structuring of my personal temporality resonates around present conscious concerns, with both past and future synthesized in the relational focus of my preoccupying activity of the moment.

That process we call memory is all too often conceived of in the simplest of terms, without appropriate attention paid to its connection with the present. It would be a disservice to merely note that memory is a recollection of events which occurred prior to now. To make such a claim would be to deny the creatively active role of consciousness, thereby reducing memory to a passive replaying of all events recorded, as it were, on the mind of those who had earlier experienced what now appears as memory. That an event occurred is most often not debatable, what its significance *was* or *is*, is most certainly open to question. In short, the past like all other facts is incapable of speaking for itself; it is continually being reconstructed. A similar fate would lie in store for the *NOW*, since before it could be grasped it would instantly be memory. If we step away from a mechanistic perspective, concentrating instead on time as experience, it is possible to achieve a better understanding of the unity of past, present and future as dimensions of our experiential sense of duration. To phrase the issue another way, all three are reconstructed out of our intentionality, not existing merely as points on a temporal line, but as contingencies whose horizons are perpetually shifting around the constitutive concerns of the moment (Husserl, 1964).

In what we term memory there is not merely a random appearance of events emerging out of the fog of the past, nor is there a complete retrieval of "data" from the brain's "memory bank." It is fair to say, to be remembered, events must be recognized as relevant to some or other project. While it is true we do have what may be termed incidental memories, events remembered but not consciously recalled until probing brings them forth, even these are apparently related to intentional memories, the salient features of which evolve out of present attention. Precisely where *NOW* leaves off and memory enters the picture is always unclear, as the delineation of each is made in terms of relevant frames of reference. In a seminal discussion of this interaction of present and past, James (1890) pointed out that *NOW* is a specious moment, a useful fiction not to be found. In fact, he preferred to think of *NOW* as a "saddle back" which we sit astride looking to the immediate past and future in order to gain our orientation in time. Whitehead (1957), commenting on the same puzzle as to the existence of the present, claims "What we perceive as present is a vivid fringe of memory tinged with anticipation . . . the past and the future meet and mingle in the ill-defined present."

The thrust of James' remarks has been made by others as well, we do not live our lives in a series of desultory moments unconnected in either direction. Experiencing itself is a time-creating activity, which, depending on the project at hand, synthesizes past, present and future through a sense of duration and anticipation (Heidegger, 1970). A graphic ilustration of part of the process may be seen in Figure 2.

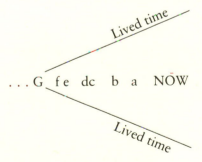

Figure 2. Memory and Experiental Time.

NOW exists as an extended moment or field wherein consciousness is directed by a particular task back to the salient memory, *G*--one which is linked by the focus of consciousness to *NOW*. Analytically *NOW* is less real than it is experientially since it is in a constant state of flux. Nonetheless, the *NOW* of consciousness has an existence in time, akin if you will, to the existence of a body in space. The exact dimensions of *NOW* are designated by the successive tasks of attention. Whatever the intervening events represented by *a* through *f* might be they are largely ignored, unseen by the mind's eye. It is as if there were an intentional arc whereby we reach back, reconstructing certain pertinent events, bypassing events in between, which have no significance in terms of why we delved into memory in the first place. In effect, we create a memory corridor where nothing stands out except those things implicated by momentary interests. For all intents and purposes, lived time is that period between the *NOW* of consciousness and the relevant past event. It is this sense of lived time, or what Husserl (1964) terms *duree* which constitutes the field of the specious present.

Having claimed that memory is purposive and linked to *NOW* to form a sense of duration, let me also emphasize the event "remembered" is perceived both as something past as well as something current. In structuring our temporality in terms of intentionality our experience is both continuous and episodic. Insofar as we are cognizant of some personal evolution having taken place during the span of our "lived time," we see time as stretching out behind us, as it were, and accordingly evaluate ourselves in terms of the perceived magnitude of change. In looking back we recognize some elapsed change, thereby acquiring some sense of our own personal *rate* of experience. Consequently, time appears to us to be continuous. Contemporaneously, however, we keep track of time according to the dominant focus of our attention, "grasping" it in terms of particular episodic themes. We might say that event *G* in Figure 2, marks the beginning of this particular episode and delimits one dimension of the present. It is perceived as existing, not as something once experienced, now gray with the passing of too much time. There is one nagging question which remains to be answered--how do individuals identify or "date" the interval between *NOW* and salient memory *G* which together constitute the zone of the durational present. The answer is, in any number of ways so long as they reflect socially or personally important changes. Undoubtedly some reference will be made to clock or calendar time since *G*; about three months ago, just before 7:00 o'clock or something similar. In addition, *G* may be described as having occurred in terms of some hallmarks, "before my accident" or "just as the term was beginning" or "during election week." It must be stressed that the progression of past to present is not apprehended as linear, the focus of *NOW* and the linked past *exist* together.

So far so good, but as of yet no reference has been made to the future or its role in the whole temporal process. Again it is the reflexive processes of thought which may be the key to temporal unification. To put the matter succinctly, the extensiveness of our anticipation of the future enlarges or contracts according to present intent. Like the past, the future does not simply exist, it is constructed by us and perceived as a series of expected presents. As individuals, our image of the future may involve a multiple number of time perspectives, each applicable for certain purposes, so that as we think ahead we may envision events at greater or lesser distance without any conflict in our overall temporal orientation. To be more specific, Bergson, Minkowski, James, Husserl and others contend the *NOW* is tinged with the past as well as with an anticipation of things yet to come, each suggesting in turn that there is a prefiguring of the future in our conception of the present (Sherover, 1975). In fact just as my relevant past is perceived by me as colored in terms of my present consciousness, so too does the future appear to me as an extension of the moment as already completed. Both past and future are cast, then recast, in terms of their linkage with present intent, while the time perspectives imposed on events reflect emergent values. As a consequence, no singular monolithic definition of temporality is possible. The fact that individuals manage to agree on an external measure of time in no way obviates the differential criteria employed in the creation of personal time.

For our purposes here, the stochastic relational temporal linkage between expected futures and the present moment may be labelled *prolepsis* or *proleptic imagery*.[1] In effect, we "recollect the future," in much the same manner as we reconstruct the past--in an epochal relationship to the *NOW* of experience--as a forward extension of what already is. Our conception of the future is the antecedent of it, residing in the present. In either case the concerns of the *NOW* are the operative element organizing our temporal orientation (Luhmann, 1976). Turning to Figure 3, the left side duplicates what was presented previously, that is, to the right of *NOW* lies our anticipated future. As can be seen, the extentiveness of the orientation depicted is postulated to be roughly equivalent to the length or depth of the salient retrospective time track. In essence, the future may be thought of as the operationalization of the transcendant concerns of the present, just as the past is also reconstituted by its intentionality.

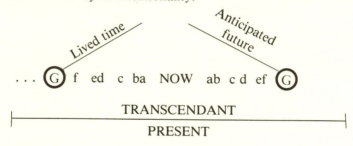

Figure 3. Temporal extension of the Present.

In no way should the graphic presentation be taken as evidence that time is indeed a linear progression or that there is an exact symmetry of past and future. The intervals depicted are neither uniform nor equal, rather they are but an imperfect way to suggest the existence of orienting issues which shape the continuity of time tracks and denote the beginning, end and future extension of current projects. (For a general discussion, see Lyman and Scott, 1970.) As durational beings our sense of what is *present* encompasses the further reaches of the particular track brought into mind by the question at hand; it is not bounded by the immediacy of clock time. Of course, the role played in this whole process by the age of the actor cannot be ignored; except for accounting for the density of prior experience and a possible foreshortening of future orientation, the basic relationship should continue to operate.

A METHODOLOGICAL APPROACH TO TIME IN MIND

If standard chronological measures of temporal processes are of limited utility for grasping the lived times of experience, what alternatives are there? One analytic tool which should prove invaluable for describing the interplay of diverse temporal tracks is what has been called the sociological calendar. As a means of capturing the very socially defined units of time which structure the times of our lives, this device focuses precisely on the question of the most powerful themes and critical dates organizing our temporal horizons. As originally developed by Renee Fox (1957) notes that time analyzed in terms of its socially significant meanings allows the sociologist to ". . .reverse the priorities between action and time; that is . . . to discover the natural units of time latent in a social event or series of actions." In addition it enables attention to be directed to nature, pace and "interconnected phases of social processes," rather than the separation inherent in Julian-based descriptions. Light goes on to point out how the sociological calendar concentrates on the experiential dimensions of time as it is conceived by the actors involved, thus revealing the interrelationship between diverse realms of existence which might not otherwise be apparent.

Analytically, the units identified by a sociological calendar reflect the rhythm and change of pressing issues and pacesetting activities. In the case of medical students, Light describes how the students' conception of the phases of their training is only tangentially related to the manifest divisions of the academic calendar. Instead of four years or eight semesters, the phases of their medical school experience are seen as unfolding in five stages, each of which is characterized by a dominant perspective. Students' passage from one to the next stage is noted not only by a change in their responsibilities, but in their attitudes as well. According to Light, the internal tempo of the stages is uniquely reflective of the exigencies encountered in each as well as by the primary attitudinal focus of those undergoing passage. Although the sociological calendar has yet to be fully developed, its use has been limited thus far to one set of issues at a time, it suggests a viable avenue for analyzing the constitution of the multiple temporal reckoning systems found in the life world. The issues discussed here are obviously quite controversial, the debate being waged in their behalf is long-standing as the questions are quite complex; no simple resolution is likely to be forthcoming insofar as intentionality is a thematic characteristic of the definition of temporal episodes, the sociological calendar promises to enhance sociology's ability to adequately represent how the ebb and flow of social time is actually experienced in its many guises.

[1]Prolepsis, literally, is to take beforehand or to think in the future perfect tense, where a future act is apprehended as already accomplished in order to structure behavior toward that goal. The idea of anticipated presents is familiar in much of the phenomenological literature. Heidegger's "anticipatory resoluteness" (1970) is similar though he implies an almost teleologic linkage as we live toward our potentiality-for-Being, thereby circumscribing our immediate present and futures accordingly. Nevertheless, time ahead-of-itself has the character of "having been" and thus can be conceived of as a guide for proceding.

What this does to the usual criteria for temporal ordering in cause and effect relationships in the realm of human action is a topic appropriate for a separate discussion. However, it should be evident that the thrust of the motion of prolepsis calls for a reevaluation of the conception of *conditiones sine quibus non* as the affectors of behavior. What Thomas Reid and others critique as the "active power" in discussions of causality is implicitly a positivist-based causal model which ultimately may be inappropriate for the subject matter of sociology.

My own thoughts on this issue have profited from discussions with my colleague Lawrence Busch. They are being incorporated in a manuscript in progress entitled *Time in Social Science: Issues of Relevance.*

REFERENCES

Aristotle. *Physics.* Translated by R. Hope. Lincoln: University of Nebraska Press, 1961.

Augustine. *Confessions.* Translated by V.J. Burke. New York: Fathers of the

Church, 1953.

Berger, P. *Facing Up To Modernity*. New York: Basic Books Inc., Publishers, 1977.

Bergson, H. *Duration and Simultaneity*. Translated by L. Jacobsen. Indianapolis: Bobbs-Merrill Co., Inc., 1965.

Bock, P.K. "Social Time and Institutional Conflict," *Human Organization* 25, 2 (1966), pp. 96-102.

Braudel, F. "History and the Social Sciences," in *Economy and Society*. Ed. by P. Burke. New York: Harper & Row, 1972, pp. 11-42.

Cope, L. "Calendars of the Indians North of Mexico," *University of California Publications in American Archaeology and Ethnology,* 16, 4 (1919), pp. 119-176.

Durkheim, E. *The Elementary Forms of Religious Life*. Translated by J. W. Swain. New York: The Macmillan Company, 1915.

Eddington, A.S. *The Nature of the Physical World*. Ann Arbor University of Michigan Press, 1958.

Einstein, Albert. "Autobiographical Notes," in *Problems of Space and Time*. Ed. by J.J.C. Smart. New York: The Macmillan Company, 1964.

Evans-Pritchard, E.E. *The News*. London: Oxford University Press, 1940 (1972).

Fox, R. "Training For Uncertainty," in *The Student Physician*. Ed. by R.K. Merton, G. Reader and P. Kendall. Cambridge: Harvard University Press, 1957, pp. 207-241.

Frank, L.K. "Time Perspectives," *Journal of Social Philosophy* 4 (1939), 293-312.

Gilb, Corinne Lathrop. "Time and Change in Twentieth Century Thought," *Cashiers D'Histoire Mondiale* IX, 4 (1966), pp. 867-883.

Gluckman, M. "The Utility of the Equilibrium Model in the Study of Social Change," *American Anthropologist* 70, (1968), pp. 220-237.

Halbwachs, M. *Les Cadres Sociaux De La Memoire* (The Social Framework of Memory). New York: Arno Press, 1977 (1925).

Heidegger, M. *Being and Time*. New York: Harper and Row, 1970.

Heirich, M. "The Use of Time in the Study of Social Change," *American Sociological Review* 29, 3 (1964), pp. 386-397.

Heise, David, G. Lenski and J. Wardell. "Further Notes on Technology and the Moral Order," *Social Forces* 55, 2 (1976), pp. 316-337.

Hendricks, C. Davis and Jon Hendricks. "Concepts of Time and Temporal Construction among the Aged, with Implications for Research," in *Time Roles and Self in Old Age*. Ed. by J.F. Gubrium. New York: Human Sciences Press, 1976, pp. 13-49.

Hubert, H. and M. Mauss. "Etude sommaire de la representation du temps dans la religion et la magie," Melanges d'histoire des religions. Paris: 1909. Cited in Sorokin, Sociocultural Causality, Space, Time.

Husserl, E. *The Phenomenology of Internal Time-Consciousness*. Bloomington, Indiana: Indiana University Press, 1964.

James, W. *The Principles of Psychology*. New York: Dover Books, 1950 (1890).

Johnson, R.D. "The Internal Structure of Technology," *The Sociology of Science.* Ed. by P. Halmos. Keele, England, 1972.

Light, D. "The Sociological Calendar: An Analytic Tool for Fieldwork Applied to Medical and Psychiatric Training," American Journal of Sociology, 80, 5 (March 1975), pp. 1145-1164.

Luhmann, N. "The Future Cannot Begin: Temporal Structures in Modern Societies," *Social Research* 43, 1 (1976), pp. 130-152.

Lyman, S. and M. Scott *A Sociology of the Absurd.* New York: Appleton-Century-Crofts, 1970.

Maltz, D.N. "Primitive Time-Reckoning As A Symbolic System," *Cornell Journal of Social Relations* 3, 2 (1968), pp. 85-112.

Mannheim, Karl. *Essays on the Sociology of Knowledge.* Ed. by P. Kecskemet. London: Routledge & Pegan Paul, 1952.

Maxwell, R.J. "Anthropological Perspectives," in *The Future of Time.* Ed. by H. Osmond and F. Cheek. Garden City, New York: Anchor Books, 1971, pp. 36-72.

Mumford, Lewis. *Technics and Civilization.* New York: Harcourt, Brace & World, Inc., 1934.

Nillson, M.P. *Primitive Time Reckoning.* Lund: C.W.K. Gleerup, 1920.

Rezsohazy, R. "The Concept of Social Time: Its Role in Development," *International Social Science Journal* 24, 1972, pp. 26-36.

Sherover, C.M. *The Human Experience of Time.* New York: New York University Press, 1975.

Smart, J.J.C. "Time," in *The Encyclopedia of Philosophy.* Ed. by P. Edwards. New York: Macmillan Publishing Co., Inc. and The Free Press, 1967, pp. 126-134.

Sorokin, P.A. and Robert K. Merton. "Social Time: A Methodological and Functional Analysis," *The American Journal of Sociology* XLII, 5 (1937), pp. 615-629.

Sorokin, P.A. *Sociocultural Causality, Space, Time.* New York: Russell & Russell, Inc., 1964.

Stevens, R. "Spatial and Temporal Models in Husserl's IDEEN II," *Cultural Hermeneutics* 3, 2 (1975), pp. 105-117.

Tiryakian, E.A. "The End of an Illusion and the Illusion of the End," paper presented to American Sociological Association, Chicago, September, 1977.

Whitehead, A.N. *The Concept of Nature.* Ann Arbor, Mich.: Ann Arbor Books, 1957, p. 73. Quoted in R.G. Burton, "The Human Awareness of Time: An Analysis," *Philosophy and Phenomenological Research* XXXVI, 3 (1976), pp. 303-318.

Whitrow, G.J. *The Natural Philosophy of Time.* London: Thomas Nelson & Sons Ltd., 1961.

_____. *The Nature of Time.* New York: Holt, Rinehart and Winston, 1972.

Williams, D.C. "Myth of Passage." *Journal of Philosophy* 48 (1951), pp. 457-472.

Woodcock, G. "The Tyrany of the Clock," *Politics* 3 (1944), pp. 265-267.

LOPATA: How do you handle the fact that we redefine the world? Let's say an event occurs. We then compress and re-structure in memory. In the women that I've been interviewing the birth, for example, of a second or third child will restructure the time from marriage to the birth of the first child.

HENDRICKS: That's exactly what I was trying to indicate be-fore. Maybe you have said it better than I have--that there's an intentional arc, and if I ask you to remember something out of the blue, likely as not you'll say, "In what realm?" My response is that the temporal dimension of the woman remembering the birth of a child is very much different than the one remembering her own high school graduation or her own intellectual develop-ment. The intervals necessary to measure that change should change accordingly and not be referred back to science or a standard. That's the idea of a sociological calendar, as Rene Fox had in 1957 and Donald Light published in an article in *AJS*, March 1975.

V. MARSHALL: I'd like to comment on the relation between the lived time and the anticipated future. You seem to suggest there was a balance struck, as measured in social time units of some sort. My own data, and I give myself quite a bit of freedom in interpreting it, show that there is a relationship in-deed, but not a balancing one. Ask old people, average age 80, how long they anticipate living--that sets an outer boundary on anticipated future. What you find, roughly speaking, is when people begin to see that boundary as real, as getting close to it, a process like what Butler called the life reviews occurs and they start filling in A, B, C, D, E, F in lived time, retrospection, or in memory. The longer this process of the review continues, the more events they will fill in. In other words, it takes time to build the story of their lives as a series of significant events. I get this by asking people, "I'd like you to tell me the major turning points of your life." The longer the review goes on, the more turning points they will give. When the past gets built or re-constructed in the life review process you get a past time per-spective--people are focusing more on the past, and you get a re-striction of futurity in terms of measures of how far ahead you plan your future. Once that process appears to be completed, or if it's completed, if people live that long, next comes a shifting away from the past, and the anticipated future is extended in terms of how far ahead people will plan, but there are fewer A, B, C, D, E's and F's than that. These people literally keep a calendar where they list events that they want to do, vacations that they want, and so forth, but it is less intense--further ahead in time, but less planned.

HENDRICKS: I don't think we contradict. What I am saying here is that instead of asking people how long they have to live, ask, "How different will you be when you die than you are now." Suppose a person who retired five years ago is saying, "Between retirement and now I've changed thus and so, and between now and death I'll probably change about the same amount." If you shift the focus and say, "How different are you from the time of the birth of your child till now," which extends the focal length a great deal more, these events will assume even less significance and G will stretch back in time. Then ask them to project ahead. You'll find that the magnitude of change is extended even though in calendar time it's still five years. What I'm saying is these things are both horizons--mental constructs that we use depending on our purpose at hand. I'm just saying that the depth of the future time perspective is a reflection of the depth of the past time perspective.

MIZRUCHI: I want to briefly convey an idea from the gerontology conference at Vichy on the same subject: Time takes smaller steps during old age. I think that's what Vic is getting at, and that's compatible with what you're saying, except that this is abstracted from structural conditions or situational conditions in which we are thrust. There is a qualitative dimension associated with generational consciousness.

SCHWARTZ: What you have there is a set of elements organized in the form of a queue. A queue, of course, consists of tasks organized in terms of priority. In one respect, a calendar is a queue because it involves a set of tasks or obligations organized in terms of priority--one thing to be done before the other. Our appointment books contain a set of queued tasks or obligations. One of the characteristics of aging, I think, is that the queue becomes smaller. There are fewer demands on the time of the individual and as a result the past becomes denser in terms of demands per time unit. So the sense of boredom is to be characterized by the absence of a queue to administer or a calendar which is empty. It seems to me that you have presented a model for the analysis of time conceptions which could be used to differentiate people at different points in their life cycles. Indeed, the imagery of your diagram is the imagery of a queue. I would therefore alter that diagram by putting the A's, B's and C's on the left-hand side a bit closer together, and add more letters. But the letters on the right-hand side, among the aged, would be fewer and more scattered. We were talking at breakfast about the fact that despised and/or dependent groups, like children and old people, tend to be characterized as having a surplus of time whereas the productive groups in our society are characterized in the opposite sense. It seems to me that what I've said, and what other people have said in the seminar, is quite consistent with that idea. Of course, time surplus and scarcity and self-conception or identity are closely tied together, since the value of one's time and the value of one's self are really two aspects of the same thing. Value of self and the concept of time scarcity can be conceptualized with the queuing model of the life cycle.

HENDRICKS: I agree that your queuing model is very similar.

GLASSNER: First, to pick up on a point regarding the number of letters on each side. In my research with manic depressives, it struck me immediately that in their depressive phase there are a lot of A's through Z's for past, but very few future events; whereas in the manic phase it's exactly the opposite--a lot of letters for the future and few for the past. Secondly, I can't help but comment on the operationalization you did because it strikes me that you're specifying time for your respondents, and I just have to say that that's unfortunate.

HENDRICKS: I share your feeling, but I'm not sure the quandary is resolvable.

GLASSNER: I'm not sure it's operationalizable in that sense. Then thirdly, to back up to something way back in the presentation, you bring up the interesting point that we have universal temporal symbols such as clocks and calendars. If they're here to stay, then Newton is sort of saved, because the problems for Newtonian Time have been: Who looks, and what do they look at? If we can solve that with universal symbols, then Newton is somewhat saved.

HENDRICKS: I don't mind saving him, but I don't want to canonize him in the process.

GLASSNER: It struck me that we have an interesting cycle there if, in fact, we have a global community with these symbols.

HENDRICKS: I think the temporal symbol of the clock now is probably the only thing that cuts across the various forms of organizing these other levels--different kinds of industrial societies, different kinds of social settings. I think that's the sole symbol we have left, but it does provide a synthesis. I think, in terms of personal experience, the sole synthesis we have left is this one: experience, consciousness.

BEATTIE: I think Barry Schwartz was talking about older people having more open or unstructured time. I have some concern that we don't automatically make assumptions about all older persons when we have such tremendous heterogeneity. I don't think we really have addressed the question of the perceptions of time among the older population and whether it is less structured institutionally in the traditions of work or family, but we may have other kinds of structures that certain groups in the aging population may be dealing with but others may not. I think you'll find this in some our our work here in Syracuse.

HENDRICKS: I agree completely and brought along another published paper that appeared in the Gubrium book on time roles and self in old age. I'm agreeing with you.

CAIN: In addition to the queues or the multiple formats, we need to add another complexity. The individual may carry multiple definitions of his or her own age at a given time. Very specifically, I had an interview with an ex-convict a few years ago. He was approximately age 40 and had been in prison about half of his life, and I had noticed that among other things he had a young woman around his arm in recent weeks. I was asking him why and he paused and said, "You know, when I walked out of that prison a few months ago, I was at least three

separate ages at the same time. For purposes of a boy-girl, relationship," he said, "I'm still a teenager. I have not known girls,
been with a girl in contact, since my childhood." About a week
ago I had a prisoner serving a triple life sentence who had been
paroled and he said, "I'm 45 years old, but in terms of
chronological age, I'm 17." But he said that he'd been working
for months and months before getting out, trying to adjust and
dress in a business suit. He knew he was about 40 and had to be
a middle-aged person, and present himself to an employer. But
then he said, also, that he had essentially become old--he felt
himself to be an old man during those last years in prison. "No
wonder I'm confused." he said.

Chapter **2** # TIME AS A TOOL FOR POLICY ANALYSIS IN AGING

Thomas Pastorello, Ph.D.
School of Social Work
Syracuse University

Recently, in the pages of *The American Sociological Review,* a three-year debate on the "futile quest" of statistical attempts to separate age, period and cohort effects, culminated in a comment by Norval Glenn (1976:900):

The great bulk of the literature on cohort analysis is devoted to methods or attempts to separate statistically age, period and cohort effects. The effects are named for the kinds of influences which produce them; age effects are produced by influences associated with the aging process, period effects by influences associated with each period of time and cohort effects by influences associated with membership in each birth cohort. Regardless of how cohort data are examined, two kinds of effects are confounded with one another, age and cohort effects are confounded in cross-sectional data by age, age and period effects in intra-cohort trend data, and period and cohort effects in trend data for each age level. . . *a strictly statistical solution to the age-period-cohort problem is not possible. . .* mechanical, atheoretical cohort analysis depends at least as much on knowledge of *theories of aging* and of recent history as on technical expertise. (Emphasis mine.)

Were statisticians and sociologists, reading this and similar messages in the literature, to turn immediately to us gerontologists for expertise on "theories of aging," we would find ourselves in an embarassing position. Lacking comprehensive

46

theory in social gerontology, we too are at a loss to make sense out of life course data which invariably confound the time effects of age (or maturation), period (or time of measurement) and cohort. It is, therefore, the purpose of this paper to set forth a heuristic set of concepts, in the form of a time-based paradigm, as a step toward the building of comprehensive theory in aging -- theory which would enable us to adequately analyze life course data and, consequently, develop a rational scheme for research-based planning and policy aging.

Although "aging" is a basic temporal concept, time as a conceptual tool for theory building in social gerontology has not been systematically employed. This paucity of temporal concepts exists despite the fact that as early as 1943 Sorokin, in his seminal work on socio-cultural time, introduced a host of concepts which, when modified, I believe show promise for systematic application in life course studies. [1] The temporal concepts are sequence, duration, rate, rhythm, recurrence, routine and synchronization. These concepts, in conjunction with the other temporal concepts of age, period and cohort, and my method for the integration of the concepts, constitute the paradigm I have developed. (See Diagram 1.) The paradigm is put forth as a set of procedures for the unconfounding of time effects in life course data by means of an integration of research methodology with time-based theory in sociology and social gerontology. [2] The utility of the paradigm, as a research-based policy tool, will be demonstrated in this paper by its application to an understanding of the retirement problem.

Diagram 1

Time Paradigm

Antecendents	Socialization-Allocation	Consequences
Cohort (Age differences)	Synchronization	Individual (Roles)
History (Period effects)	Asynchronization	Sequence
Maturation (Age change)		Duration
		Rate
		Individual and Organizational
		Rhythm
		Recurrence
		Routine

The key integrating concept of the paradigm is synchronization. Social change is viewed partially as a function of the degree of synchronization or asynchronization[3] between socialization and allocation processes. (Socialization is defined as the learning of expectations and behaviors relevant to roles and positions acquired throughout the life span, and allocation as the distribution of roles and positions throughout social structure.[4]) The "retirement problem" (to the extent that it is a problem) may be offered as an example of how the paradigm may be applied in policy-relevant research. The retirement role is one the allocation of which is often mandatory. Its allocation, however, is not well synchronized with the socialization processes leading up to retirement, in that extensive and thorough preparation programs for retirement do not exist. This is a type of macrosociological asynchronization.

The *antecedents* of synchronization/asynchronization may be understood in terms of historical (period or time-of-measurement effects), demographic (cohort effects) and maturational perspectives (age effects). In understanding the consequences of synchronization/asynchronization, the paradigm employs the set of time concepts described by Sorokin as sequence, duration and rate (which I apply to and define in terms of individual role phenomena), and rhythm, recurrence and routine (which may be extended to the phenomena of organizational activity).

To extend the example on the "problem" of retirement, one may seek an understanding of retirement - asynchronization's antecedents in terms of *demographic, historical,* and *maturational* "explanations." For example, lack of societal preparation for retirement may be understood in terms of the baby boom cohort's exertion of increasing pressure for jobs (deficient allocation), thereby forcing mandatory retirement with little time for planning preparatory programs. This is a short-based, or *demographic,* "explanation." Of course, there is an *historical* argument often put forth: rapid technological change has made and is making the knowledge possessed by older workers increasingly obsolete. Early, unwanted retirement may be seen as one consequence of this trend. It is very important to note, for reasons to be emphasized later that, perhaps, *maturational* trends least plausibly explain early, unwanted retirement -- at least to the extent that physical and mental health remain adequate for employment well into advanced old age for many aging individuals.

The paradigm dictates that we also explore the possible consequences of retirement-related asynchronization. The cohort antecedent explanation for early retirement, which also helps explain later entry into the job market on the part of young people (extended adolescence), has consequences for the *duration* of life course work related roles. The predicted trend is for the length of careers to be shortened. To the extent that technological change makes knowledge and skills increasingly obsolete (the historical antecedent explanation), the career line *sequence* of promotions is interrupted, with the very top statues being eliminated for many individuals. *Rate* of movement through the promotion sequence is, of course, slowed.

On the social structural level, change in the duration of the work cycle has consequences for the overall *rhythm* of social life, with significant social phenomena, e.g., the average age of entry into the job market, occuring at different times. *Routines* within the institutions of education, work and leisure must, as a consequence, adjust. To the extent that a period of extended adolescence fosters adolescents' looking for temporary job opportunities before permanently entering the job market and to the extent that workers begin to prepare for early retirement, increasing their present levels of leisure time and education; periods of work, education and recreation are likely to *recur* throughout the life course rather than remain in their present fixed sequence of education, work and recreation-leisure (retirement).

I have applied this type of analysis to asynchronization problems related to roles less formally allocated and socialized than the retirement role, e.g., the leisure participant role among American elderly. Time does not permit me to continue with examples; however, I hope that I have demonstrated that application of the time concepts of the paradigm leads us to the organization of different, and often complementary, explanations and understanding of aging phenomena. Of course, the basic principles of theory building must be applied to choose among them or state the need for additional explanations.

By contributing to theory building in social gerontology, the Time Paradigm also contributes to a solution of the problem of confounded age, cohort and history effects. As noted previously, even the most sophisticated analysis of variance procedures (Schaie, 1965) succeed in unconfounding only two of the three time effects for any given analysis. For example, Schaie's time sequential model offers a net age effect, a net period effect, but leaves us to make the assumption that cohort differences are theoretically unimportant. Likewise, his cohort-sequential and cross-sequential models force the researcher to assume the unimportance of historical effects and age effects, respectively. When these models for data analysis are applied blindly, i.e., atheoretically, results are uninterpretable. The Time Paradigm, however, stipulates that within any set of complementary or alternative explanation for a given asynchronization-related aging phenomenon, at least one explanation be put forth based on maturational age changes, one explanation be put forth based on cohort differentials and one explanation be put forth based on historical changes. An assessment of the theoretical plausibility of each explanation would then aid in the choice among time-sequential, cohort-sequential, or cross-sequential methodological strategies. In the brief example on retirement given previously, the maturational explanation seemed the least plausible. That datum alone would call for use of a cross-sequential model for analysis. At the level of antecedents, therefore, the paradigm fosters the integration of theory and methods in social gerontology.

At the paradigmatic level of *consequences*, integrated theory and methods is established as a firm base for policy and planning in aging. Despite the connotations of terms used to describe the Time Paradigm, the system implied in the paradigm is recursive and allows for causal flow from the variables listed under "consequences" to the variable listed under "antecedents." Any theoretical model has policy relevance to the extent that the variables its concepts imply are manipulable.

In the past, legislation has affected the duration of roles and positions, the sequence in which they are taken on, and the rate at which individuals are allowed to move through an entire sequence. In this regard, consider the impact of selective service legislation, mandatory education laws, and compulsory retirement laws on the temporal aspects of role performance. In the future, theoretical understanding of the mutual effects of one Time Paradigm variable on another, or one set of Time Paradigm variables on another, could guide legislation toward the goal of adjusting the temporal aspects of role performance in a manner which compensates for macro-sociological asynchronization. Does not mandatory retirement legislation presently attempt to do just that? The goal of policy derived from informational analyses based on the Time Paradigm would be, therefore, the facilitation of social and personal adjustment by the elderly to the problems of retirement, widowhood and leisure, related to asynchronization between allocation and socialization processes.

The "consequences" aspect of the Time Paradigm facilitates policy making in aging, or rational choice among alternative directives for the attainment of specific objectives in life course planning, by offering a common conceptual language with which alternative directives, from a diversity of perspectives, can be rephrased and, therefore, more readily compared. This is true in that temporal conceptual schemes are implicit in all modes of policy analysis in the area of aging.

A brief and necessarily limited examination of policy proposals in the area of aging, disseminated by the Center for Policy Process (1977), will now be made for the purpose of demonstrating the utility of the Time Paradigm as an evaluative model for the assessment of policy alternatives in terms of their likely impact on individuals and social structure. The five proposals I will discuss share as their basic goal the bringing about of a more personally and socially beneficial use of work, education and leisure throughout the life course.

The Julie M. Sugarman plan proposes that workers be allowed a sabbatical every 10 years, to be financed by annual 6% payroll deductions. Such a plan would help make more cyclic the traditional linear sequence of education, work and leisure (retirement) roles by allowing for more education and leisure than normally acquired during the work years. Extended would be the duration of education-and leisure-related roles, but the rate at which one moves through the work-devoted segment of the lifespan would be little affected. A new routine would be introduced into the organization of work were this system widely adopted. Sabbaticals would recur every 10 years for individuals but would have to be planned for by management on a continual basis. The total result may very well be the imposition of a new rhythm on organizational life and on career span activity -- much in the same way that holidays declared during the 20th Century imposed a new rhythm on the work year. This new rhythm would approximate and, therefore, facilitate the integration of socialization and allocation processes.

Because those on sabbatical may use their time off for any purpose, the potential for retraining to deal with knowledge absolescence in one's job is an important possibility to consider. The opportunity for retraining would facilitate socialization to the work role during the latter half of the work span -- a time during which lack of continued socialization may lead to lower job satisfaction and self-esteem because of the rapid pace of technological change in most industries. The potential also exists for use of the one year for general education and other leisure pursuits. The use of time in this manner would facilitate anticipatory socialization to retirement by periodically offering lengthly periods of free time to workers before retirement. Such acclimation periods may prove to be very important for the restructuring of free time as leisure time during the last 1/3 of the life span. Socialization-allocation synchronization would be facilitated to the extent that workers become better prepared for the retirement role when it is formally allocated.

Gosta Rehn has proposed a public insurance system based on transfer of income among different periods of life of the individual. Each individual would be credited with an account containing a specific amount of funds to cover unemployment, welfare, education and pension needs during his or her life time and the account may be drawn upon to cover extended periods of "creative non-employment."

The Rehn public insurance, transfer of income system would contribute to a cyclic modification of the traditional linear sequence of education, work and leisure roles. Under this plan, however, greater control would be extended over the duration of education and leisure roles and over the rate at which one moves through the work-devoted segment of the life span than under the Sugarman plan. Within the resources of the insurance fund, one is free to take leaves of absence from work for periods of time greater than or less than one year and at frequencies greater than or less than every 10 years. In addition, to the extent that one conserves funds, drawings on the pension fund may begin earlier than at the traditional retirement age, and, therefore, lead to a shortening of the work span. To the extent that one makes liberal use of the leave-of-absence provisions, retirement *per se* may be indefinitely postponed, therefore, lengthening the work span while at the same time probably increasing job satisfaction.

This plan would also introduce a new routine into the organization of work; however, because the recurrence of leaves is based on individual decision, the rhythm imposed on organizational activity will be more erratic and less predictable than that imposed by the Sugarman plan. The ability of management to plan and compensate for leaves would be taxed and, consequently, the feasibility of the Rehn plan is to be seriously challenged. Like the Sugarman plan, Rehn's proposed insurance system facilitates socialization-allocation synchronization in regard to work adjustment during the latter parts of the work span and in regard to retirement and the use of leisure time. However, the Sugarman plan would be more likely than the Rehn plan to improve work allocation to those seeking part-time employment or apprenticeships. This may prove to be the case because given its greater rhythmic predictability, the Sugarman plan facilitates hiring and training plans aimed at the unemployed needed to take the place of those on leave. Of the two, therefore, the Sugarman plan better integrates socialization-allocation processes in regard to work training.

The Santa Clara County "Cafeteria Plan" allows workers

to trade in percentages of their income (up to 20%) for time off from work in addition to vacation (up to two 21-day periods during one year). This plan seems more restrictive than either the Sugarman or Rehn plans in that work, education and leisure role sequences become modifiable only within a one-year cycle. Control over the duration of leisure-related roles is minimal and the rate at which one moves through the work-devoted segments of the life span is unaffected.

This plan too introduces a new routine into the organization of work; however, the recurrence of leaves is more predictable than under the Rehn plan. The "Cafeteria Plan" does not so much impose a new rhythm of work year already established by existing holidays and traditional vacation allowances. Like the Sugarman plan it facilitates work allocation to those seeking part-time jobs because of its predictability. However, because leave periods are short in duration under the "Cafeteria Plan," the plan is not likely to create much work, nor is it likely to create opportunities for apprenticeships. Of the three, this plan is probably least likely to facilitate lifetime socialization-allocation synchronization. Because the worker is very aware of the fact that he or she has traded in income for free time, that time is not likely to be used for voluntary job re-training. Use of the free time for leisure pursuits is probable but, nevertheless, not likely to socialize or prepare one for retirement, in that blocks of time larger than 21 days would be necessary to simulate retirement and, therefore, acclimate one to retirement.

The Marziale Flexible Retirement Plan is one which allows older workers the option of combining a partial pension plan with part-time or reduced work hours. Unlike the other plans, this one does not call for significant modification of the linear sequence of education, work and leisure (retirement) life-time roles. It places its emphasis, rather, on shortening the duration of work-related roles, lengthening the duration of retirement and leisure related roles and modifying the rate at which one moves through the work-devoted segment of the life span by allowing for a gradual movement into retirement.

Routine within the organization of work is affected little. What change in individual routine that may occur will be largely experienced by older cohorts of workers as they begin to work less hours of time weekly. The major event which the Marziale Plan facilitates, gradual retirement, is not a recurrent phenomenon. The other three plans do stress recurrent phenomena with their emphasis on leaves and vacations. Therefore, the rhythm of organizational life is changed little by the Marziale Plan. The down beat between work and retirement is, however, more subdued. The Marziale Plan is explicitly designed to facilitate socialization-allocation synchronization in regard to retirement. The gradually decreasing period of part-time work between full-time work and retirement creates a social condition which is very likely to increase the success of pre-retirement socialization. The gradual increase of free time allows workers to test out leisure roles and pursue further education and, therefore, make better use of free time when it arrives in abundance during retirement. Because large blocks of part-time work will be freed-up by older workers in a highly predictable manner, the plan should improve the allocation of jobs to those seeking part-time work or apprenticeships in various industries.

Interestingly, this plan facilitates socialization-allocation synchronization in regard to retirement without introducing a notion of cyclic life planning, i.e., the linear sequence of education, work and leisure roles is not tampered with. However, the Marziale Plan's failure to introduce a mechanism to vary the sequence of these lifetime roles limits its utility in the area of socialization-allocation synchronization in regard to work. The increase in free time offered by this plan occurs at a stage in the career span when this time's use for job-retraining or career change would be unlikely. Therefore, the Marziale Plan also suffers in comparison to the Sugarman plan.

Fred Best and Barry Stern, researchers also doing work in the area of life course planning, do not offer one specific proposal for the life-time redistribution of education, work and leisure; rather, they argue that any plan which incorporates cyclic life planning will simultaneously deal with many problems related to education, work and leisure. As the previous analyses of the four specific proposals, using the Time

Paradigm, indicates, this is not necessarily the case. The Rehn Public Insurance Plan is limited in its ability to allocate part-time work and apprenticeships in spite of its cyclic nature, and the feasibility of its implementation is limited because of it. The Santa Clara Plan is also limited in its work allocation features despite its cyclic aspects and, in addition, does not contribute to job-retraining, career change or socialization to retirement. Further, the Marziale Flexible Retirement Plan shows a potential for facilitating socialization to retirement despite the fact that it does not incorporate a cyclic life plan.

The basic problem with the Best and Stern model is that it does not explicitly incorporate temporal dimensions beyond a concern with role "sequence." The Time Paradigm sketched out in this document explicitly incorporates the temporal dimensions of "duration," "rated," "routine," "recurrence," "rhythm," and "synchronization" as well as "sequence" for policy analysis in the field of aging. In addition, it incorporates the temporal dimensions of "age," "cohort" and "time-of-measurement" to improve the quality of empirical research used as a basis for policy development.

The application of the Time Paradigm for the comparative analysis of the Sugarman, Rehn, Santa Clara County and Marziale proposals leads to the conclusion that the directives embodied in the Sugarman proposal are most likely to lead to the attainment of aging policy objectives related to work, education and leisure (retirement). The Time-based Paradigm offered a conceptual language which facilitated the comparison of these proposals. It contains dimensions in the areas of policy research methodology, policy consequences for individual role-related behavior, policy consequences for organizational structure and change, and policy-facilitating theory for understanding policy consequences for problems relating to the socialization to and allocation of educational, occupational and leisure roles and opportunities. Lest policy analysis be as limiting as the one the Best and Stern model provides, a tool for policy analysis need be at least as comprehensive as the Time Paradigm. The ultimate goal of the further work proposed to be done in the development of the time paradigm is, therefore, nothing less

important than a contribution to the science of policy making
for and with the elderly.

FOOTNOTES

[1] An important conceptualization of social time, distinct from chronological
time, stems from Sorokin's understanding of sociocultural time (1943). Chronological time, or the time of classical mechanics, according to Sorokin, is continuous, infinitely divisible, uniformly flowing, purely quantitative, and devoid of
any qualities. On the other hand, sociocultural time conceives and measures sociocultural phenomena - their duration, synchronicity, sequence, and change - in
terms of other sociocultural phenomena taken as the point of reference. It does
not flow evenly in the same group and in different societies. The moments of sociocultural time are uneven and contain eventful and critical moments as well as
stretches of empty duration. Sociocultural time is not infinitely divisible.
Sorokin notes the example of renting a room: it may be rented for a month, a
week, a day, but rarely by the hour or the minute. Sociocultural time is qualitative and its basic function is the synchronization and coordination of social
activities in order to maintain continuity, orientation and give rhythm to social
life.

[2] At least two other viable approaches exist, I believe, to the unconfounding of
time effects in life course data. One approach would employ subjective measures
of time. Those who struggle with problems in cohort analysis do so, in part,
because the time effects are measured objectively and are, therefore mathematically interdependent. Need age be defined chronologically? Need history or period be defined as time of measurement? Need cohort be defined as time of birth?
The extent to which we are able to move away from these quantitative measures
of time, is the extent to which we will be able to break the mathematical interdependence of the measures and, therefore, approach an analysis which uncon-
founds the three basic dimensions for analytical purposes. Mannheim (1929),
for example, favors the use of subjective criteria for understanding the impact of
cohort-related phenomena and prefers the term "generation" (the "experiences
of common influences"). More important than calendar date as time of measurement (or period) is the need to know how historical events have impact on the individual, i.e., his subjective reactions. Focused interviewing would be one
method that may be employed in this regard. Finally, chronological age in many
analyses should be replaced by measures of biological, psychological or
sociological age, each of which may be weakly correlated with chronological age
and be much more appropriate theoretically.

A second approach would assume an interactive model for analysis. A given
analysis of variance model will confound one time effect (age, cohort or period)
with the other two. The same analysis offers a set of interaction effects. To the

extent that it is theoretically meaningful to view one time effect as an interaction of the other two, it would seem valid to use the interaction effect of any two time factors as an unconfounded estimate of the third. For example, it would seem reasonable to view cohort effect as the interaction of history and age for many analyses.

[3]The temporal term "asynchronization" has been applied in the field of aging before, but not in the sense that it is being applied in this work. Recently (Seltzer, 1976), the term has been applied to describe time-disordered relationships which arise when an individual's various social spheres and role-sets are not temporally synchronized. In his seminal work on life course sociology, Cain (1964) had devised this definition and wrote of its promise for sociological inquiry in the field of aging. The term, asynchronization, as developed here, is quite different. It perhaps borrows an individual, role-focused element from Cain; however, this element is merged with the macro-sociological interests of Sorokin, who viewed asynchronization as lack of coordination among social activities, to develop a social psychological concept of a synchronization as one which occurs between socialization and allocation processes.

[4]Despite Riley, Johnson and Foner's heuristic comments (1972) on the need for understanding the phasing of socialization and allocation processes, there has been no systematic attempt in social gerontology to understand the aging process as a complex temporal function of socialization and allocation process. The concepts of synchronization and asynchronization should prove to be helpful tools in this regard.

REFERENCES

Cain, Leonard D. "Life Course and Social Structure." Robert L. Faris (ed.), *Handbook of Modern Sociology,* Chicago: Rand McNally, 1964.

Center for Policy Process. Mimeographed Conference Materials: "Life Cycle Planning: New Strategies for Education, Work and Retirement in America." Conference, Washington, D.C., April, 1977.

Glen, Norval. "Cohort Analysts' Futile Quest." *American Sociological Review* 1976, (Comments), 41: 900-903.

Mannheim, Karl. "The Problem of Generations" Paul Keschemeti (ed.), (1952) *Essays on the Sociology of Knowledge,* London: Routledge and Kegan Paul, Ltd., 1929.

Riley, Matilda White; Marilyn Johnson and Anne Foner. *Aging and Society: A Sociology of Age Stratification.* New York: Russell Sage Foundation, 1972.

Schaie, K.W. "A General Model for the Study of Developmental Problems." *Psychological Bulletin,* 1963, 64:92-107.

Seltzer, Mildred. "Suggestions For The Examination of Time-disordered Relationships." Jaber F. Gubrium (ed.), *Time, Roles and Self in Old Age.*

New York: Behavioral Publishers, 1973.
Sorokin, Pitirim A. *Sociocultural Causality, Space, Time.* Durham: Duke
University Press, 1943.

HENDRICKS: In terms of benchmarks or reference points for determining synchronization, asynchronization, allocation and socialization, it seems to me you apply a career-type pattern to definable and scarcely available roles. This is fine for those roles that do have to be allocated on a finite basis. Leisure or free time roles have no such scarcity built in to them. How do you deal with leisure or free time roles within your paradigm?

PASTORELLO: I chose work-related roles in my example, but I have tried to deal with some of these other issues. I appear to give this a formal perspective, but just as Brim and Wheeler, in their work on adult socialization, talk about informal socialization, I think we can talk about informal allocation as may occur in the spontaneous generation of roles among individuals in dyads or in interaction with one another.

CAIN: I have a different problem with synchronization. My own use of the term was not in this sense at all but in the sense of not bringing a person along holistically through various stages. That is, a person may be called upon to be an adult at 16 for purposes of criminality but couldn't be an adult until 21 for purposes of signing contracts.

PASTORELLO: I see your concept of asynchronization not at the center of the paradigm but on the left side under the discussion of age. I realize you used the word asychronization in a different sense. You alluded to it earlier when you were talking about the convict who came out of jail and felt that he had three ages in some sense. Of course that obviously defies its being measured on the basis of chronological age: age measured on the basis of calendar date or time from birth.

CAIN: The problem seems to be that all socialization is anticipatory. In one sense we can anticipate formal rules, career patterns, sequence in family, and so forth. But it calls for a different conceptualization completely in anticipating unstructured roles, leisure roles. I do not see that incorporated.

HENDRICKS: That's exactly my point and one that we point out in our book. Socialization by definition is anticipatory but there are those roles in that period of life for which there are no anticipatory experiences. What then?

PASTORELLO: Don't you see Madison Avenue in a sense creating roles, allocating roles in terms of leisure pursuits in old age--what is expected of the individual in terms of leisure pursuits: riding a bike, being active, etc.?

CAIN: There's one practical question right now. I need money to deal with minority elderly. I'm trying to deal with the question of immigrants--Japanese Americans, Chinese Americans--and the question of socialization of grandparent roles on the part of the nisei when there were no role models. From where do Japanese, third generation or second generation or first generation, get their picture of old age, their picture of grandparent when there are no role models at all? So you have that type of factor as well-when you have no visible or direct historical antecedents.

V. MARSHALL: I think there's been a little left out. I think that the socialization-allocation dichotomy does in fact describe most of what has gone on in gerontological theory. In an article that should be coming out one of these years, I suggested that we may even want to do away with the notion of socialization entirely. I see glimmerings of that thought here. In this article I critique Rosow, who seems greatly disturbed because there's no role model, no motivation and so forth. If you think not just in the informal, leisure realm but in the occupational realm--if you go in ten year intervals and look at the dictionary of occupational titles, you'll find there are all kinds of new roles, if you want to call them that, being created all the time. I'm surprised that people are so upset because the same people cannot be socialized into a retirement role. Both the allocation and socialization perspectives are still tied to a notion of status position with the accompanying role. There are other theoretical approaches in sociology which are not tied to that. I tend to see both those models, in other words, as quite socially tied to a social system model in the general theory of action. They are variants on a theme of a kind of stable social system. There has been some good work there. Wilbert Moore pointed out that in a sense while human beings are mortal, societies are immortal and therefore there are all these sort of systems problems of passing people through positions, socializing people through positions and so forth, and I suppose reallocating those positions. Mannheim talks about the same problem.

Nevertheless, I think it might be fruitful at least some of the time to think just in terms of people fitting lines of activity together. There does not have to be a defined set of expectations existing for the activities of people in later life through which people must pass or into which they must be socialized. I just think we are too much tied to a status role social system model.

LOPATA: You are thinking more of functional roles?

V. MARSHALL: I'm thinking that we ought to think more in terms of a negotiated order perspective, which has the idea of people negotiating a way of life.

LOPATA: Sure. Day to day. Moment to moment, people fit their lines of activity together and they negotiate with one another and you can talk about people creating roles in process continuously and you do not have to think, at least not always, in terms of a stable set of positions through which people pass.

Chapter **3** WORK AND NON-WORK
TIME OVER THE LIFE
SPAN

Harold L. Sheppard, Ph.D.
Director, Federal Council on the Aging
Washington, D.C.

Since my topic for this conference is essentially the one of
work and time, I'd like to present some statistics concerning
work experience, first, over the past several years; and second,
among different age groups.

To begin with, the trend over the past ten years in the proportion of our 16-plus population working on a full-time basis
(35 hours or more) has changed very little, and fluctuates
according to economic conditions. For example, in 1973 -- at
the outset of the recession, 43 percent of all persons 16 and older
had worked full-time (some of them on less than a year-round
basis), but by 1976, that proportion had slipped to 41.6 percent.

On the other hand, there has been a steady increase in the
proportion working part-time on a voluntary basis, moving
from slightly more than 6 percent 10 years ago, to 7 percent last
year, 1976. We now have about 11 million Americans working
part-time on a voluntary basis -- and by voluntary I mean paid
part-time employment at the volition of the worker. That 11
million figure constitutes a 41 percent increase in 10 years in the
number of Americans working voluntarily on a part-time basis.
That 41 percent increase far exceeds the rate of increase in the
numbers working on a full-time basis, which was about 15 percent.

---

*Paper presented: Conference on the Uses of Time, Syracuse University,
November 12, 1977.

What about the figures relating to the proportion and number without any work experience at all, over this same decade? Strange as it may seem to some persons who have never looked at such data, there has been virtually no change at all. In 1966, 33.1 percent did not work; in 1976, 33.0.

When we examine the age-sex composition of the non-working population, however, there have been changes. For example, from 1966 to 1976, for all women through the age of 54, there was a decrease in the proportion with no work experience. Starting with women 55-59, the 10 year period witnessed an *increase* in the proportion without any work experience. In the case of men, there was an increase -- *regardless* of age -- in proportions without any work experience. In other words, only among women under the age of 54 was there a decrease in the proportion without any work experience. Expressing that in positive terms, in 1965 and 1976, approximately 65 percent of the *total* population 16 and older had some degree of work experience -- no change. But this lack of change in the aggregate hides the fact that *women under the age of 55 increased* in their proportions with some degree of work experience. The groups that decreased in their proportions with any work experience were, first of all, men of *all* ages, and women 55 and older.

Younger women, therefore, are moving into the work experience world, while all others -- older women, and all men, regardless of age -- are moving out.

The same data from which these remarks are derived also can provide some light on the time dimensions involved, that is, the longitudinal aspect. In 1966, for example, 52 percent of the women 25-34 years old had some degree of work experience, but 10 years later -- when we look at women 10 years older, 35-44 -- the proportion increased to 65 percent. In 1966, 56 percent of women 35-44 worked, but by the time they became 45-54, the proportion rose to 61 percent. But for women 55-59 years old in 1966, 55 percent had some work experience, and 10 years later -- when they were 65-69 -- the proportion was *lower*, only 21 percent. In other words, the retirement process among women start dramatically over the 10 year period following the age of 55.

The greatest fascination, perhaps, lies in the fact that a comparable presentation regarding men reveals that over time, regardless of which age group we start with — after the age of 24 — withdrawal from the work experience world begins. Certainly for the young male adult groups, this longitudinal decline in work experience is grounds for some interesting research, but little has been carried out to discover the possible reasons.

The fact that over a 10 year period, men 55-59 in 1966 experienced a dramatic decline work experience from 92 percent, down to 39 percent by the time they were 60-64 in 1976, comes as no surprise to gerontologists. But why the longitudinal decline in the *younger* groups of men?

Remember that I am talking about persons with absolutely no work experience at all, not even part-time for just a few weeks or so in a given year.

In this connection, I want to return to the topic of voluntary part-time employment. I mentioned earlier that the total number of persons working part-time on such a basis increased over the past decade by 41 percent. But, contrary to what many of us may have expected, the increase was preponderantly among younger persons. In the case of all Americans 45 and older, the increase was only 25 percent.

I cite this contrast because these days, there is a great deal of rhetoric concerning the utilization of older persons on a part-time basis and yet the facts are that few opportunities, apparently, have been opening up for the voluntary part-time employment of older Americans over the past 10 years. Or does this mean that such older persons are not in search of such employment — that the older adult population prefers to be using its time for full-time leisure, and is not actively seeking part-time employment? I'd better insert here the additional fact that full-time employment for this same older age group (45 and older) has increased hardly at all, by less than 3 percent — and the further fact that *in*voluntary part-time employment because of poor economic conditions increased by 39 percent from 1966 to 1976.

The overall pattern, to sum this up, is that older men and women, and younger men (under 55), are acquiring more nonwork time over the past decade. Some of this change may be considered desirable from the individual and societal standpoint, to the degree that it is voluntary. But we also know that much of it is involuntary — a result of such factors as lack of economic opportunities; a sluggish economy, involuntary retirement; and poor health.

The reduction in full-time employment, and of work experience in any amount, among older adult persons is one thing. It has meant an increase in the number of years in retirement — and on a full-time basis. But we are now undergoing a new development, namely, a decrease in mortality in the upper age groups, something that, six or seven years ago, we would not have predicted. This new development, which began about 1970, means even *more* years lived in retirement.

These factors may combine in such a way as to impinge on many of the new concepts emerging out of discussions concerning the allocation of time — especially work-time — over the life span. I refer here to the already popularized notions such as sabbaticals over the worklives of persons other than professors (or in addition to professors); of longer vacations; of reduced and flexible working hours.

You are all familiar with the myriad of new ideas and remedies now floating about among *luftmenschen* and, indeed, among responsible policy-makers. I won't detail them here. But to me they all represent, in one degree or another, a breaking up of traditional mentalities and taken-for-granted cultural forms of the distribution of work — the distribution of work in terms of (1) when, in one's lifetime, work should or might begin; (2) when, and how often, during the so-called middle years of the life span, work might be terminated and temporarily (or permanently) replaced with another form of activity; (3) how work and nonwork can be combined over a longer part of the life span than before; and (4) how, and under what conditions, permanent nonwork, i.e., fulltime retirement, might begin, and at what age. All of these dimensions, of course, would have to be tempered and modified, in accordance with the demands and possibilities flowing from type of individual, family status, occupation, and industry.

The break-up of rigid cultural forms regarding work and its timing over the life span is partly a manifestation of the belief that there is nothing instrinsic in the age of an individual — after some point of postinfancy socialization and physical development — that predetermines in rigid fashion how his or her time for work, time for learning, and time for other non-work role activities should be allocated over one's total life span — and nothing that preordains, furthermore, that one's occupation, say, after the first five years of one's regular work life, shall be a permanent, lifetime occupation.

One more "furthermore:" we are also undergoing a cultural transformation of the definition of what is meant by "old," i.e., how many years a person must be alive after birth in order to be labelled as "old." I assume that "old" will continue, for the most part, to be viewed as having negative connotations. We must be reminded that in centuries past, the number 50 was taken as the age at which persons became old.

For the past 40 years or so, 65 has been used as the chronological point, as the time point at which all work shall cease. Please don't take me too literally, but you know what I mean. To repeat the main point, we are now undergoing a transformation from 65 as that work-cessation time point to the age of 70, in the United States. I want to return to this later.

The break-up I've referred to might be seen in the many cases of young persons graduating from high school and consciously choosing to work for a while before continuing their education in college, either on a full- or part-time basis; of young persons not doing so consciously, but later on, perhaps five to 10 years later, making a decision change by entering a college or university.

At another point in the age continuum, we are witnessing dramatic adult drop-outs from full-time employment into other pursuits of a nonwork nature, perhaps on a part-time, or even a full-time basis. Other manifestations of this phenomenon take the form of sharp mid-life career changes, with which we are all familiar. I exclude from this discussion mid-life career changes brought about involuntarily by a loss of one's job, although many such career changers were simply waiting, so to speak, for a crisis of this nature to force them to make a career change about which they had fantasized for many years.

There are other forms, not typically recognized, in which the so-called linear work life formula is being violated. For example, the factory workers who make a frequent habit out of being absent on Fridays and/or Mondays — and their counterparts, the students and other single young persons who are employed in the very same factories as replacements for the regular but absent employees; or the nonproduction enterprises that hire persons of all ages during peak business weeks of the year. These persons seek such part-time work on a voluntary basis.

These remarks prompt one more possibility: We might begin to see signs of discontent and envy among *older males* (married), "Why not me, too?" "Why should others have the privilege of choice in the matter of allocation of time between work and nonwork, and not me?" When such questioning begins, we will see the full circle of the sexual revolution completed — with a more truly equal division of roles among males and females. This could involve the rotation of time-allocation to work, or a pattern of both husband and wife working at the same time, and then "leisuring" at the same time, or a pattern of both husband and wife working part-time over a number of years — depending on type of industry and occupation, individual desires, etc.

As the young of today with their acquired experience in new worktime arrangements *themselves* grow older, the probability of the extension of such arrangements over a broader life span is increased.

How much do we know of that segment of the population employed voluntarily on such a part-time, and frequently only intermittent basis?

Is this phenomenon possible only in an affluent society, by which I mean that the voluntarily part-time employed sector is not dependent solely on full-time, year-round employment for a so-called decent standard of living? Or does it portend, at least for some part of this sector, a conscious choice to reject a life-style and standard of living that can only be pursued with an income derived from year-round, full-time employment?

For the latter, the rejection means — putting it in positive terms — a deliberate preference of leisure, nonwork time over higher income-producing year-round, full-time work. Even if that choice is pursued for only a few years, and then followed by a so-called seduction into the year-round, full-time work culture, it is, nevertheless, a pattern worthy of our research and policy consideration.

I won't discuss here the notion of work sharing which, in these days of high unemployment, is receiving a great deal of policy attention — except to say that it does raise the same sociological questions I cited with regard to the voluntarily part-time employment pattern.

Finally, I must say something about the implications of the prolongation of life. Contrary to some earlier expectations and projections, of just a few years ago, we do seem to be witnessing a remarkable increase in life expectancy at the upper ages, say at 60 or 65. I won't give the precise statistics here. I refer you to the February 1977 report on vital statistics and mortality of the National Center on Health Statistics, and the ensuing Census report on new population projections into the next century, published in July 1977.

The added years that can now be expected present an extra challenge to our thinking and planning about the distribution of work over the life span, and the timing of *full and permanent retirement* from paid employment. For one thing, will we be able to continue the trend toward early retirement for increasing numbers and proportions of persons in their 60's and older — often beginning as early as the mid-50's? I refer here to (1) the capacity of the economy, and (2) the willingness of the remaining workers, to support the growing population of nonworking older persons at a level of living we ourselves would want to have, when we ourselves become eligible to join the same club.

There is such a thing as the principal of limits, and many observers believe that we are rapidly coming to the time when the limit to such a pattern has been reached. What this means, in fact, is that we may be forced to find ways of keeping people in the labor force longer than had been previously expected or planned. One of those ways, of course, is to provide meaningful part-time employment for persons in their 60's and older. Some of those persons might be the regular long-service employees of an organization; others, as new hires previously employed in other organizations.

The in-and-out-of-the-labor-force, non-linear work pattern, of course, may itself result in a postponement of full-time and permanent retirement. This certainly might be the case if a pension plan requires a certain number of equivalent full-time years in order to obtain a desired level of pension benefits.

Another implication of the prolongation of life is the increased probability that individuals will, deliberately or not, undergo significant career changes in their lives. Some of this may be the result of living long enough to be working long enough in one type of occupation to the point of becoming bored or otherwise dissatisfied with that occupation. It is not simply a coincidence, in my opinion, that over a five-year period, the middle-aged in the National Longitudinal Survey (the Parnes Study) who had *not* changed jobs experienced a decrease in job satisfaction, and that those making a voluntary job *change* experienced either an increase in satisfaction, or no decrease.

Institutional impediments aside, does such a finding mean that we should be constructing policies and programs designed to increase the pattern of mid-career changes on a more deliberate basis? And, wouldn't such policies entail, to some degree, the allocation of time to the preparation, the training and education, for such mid-career changes? Such a prospect, incidentally, is one more example of how universities, with a little imagination, might be solving some of their declining customer market problems. Instead, as you know, they are taking the typical, culture-bound solution route: Get rid of the older professors and fight the House of Representatives' bill to raise, for *all* industries, the age for mandatory retirement to 70.

GLASSNER: You were talking about the sudden decline in mortality rates since 1970. Why is that?
SHEPPARD: It is due, for the most part, to a decline in deaths

attributable to cardiovascular ailments. They speculate with some level of plausibility that this is due to the changes in our nutritional life styles, less smoking, more exercise consciousness, greater control of hypertension among men — the greatest rate of decrease has taken place among men.

HENDRICKS: The projections suggest that women are going to achieve the life expectancy, what was it, 80.6 years in the year 2000 and men about 73.

SHEPPARD: But the greatest rate of increase is taking place among men.

HENDRICKS: Are there any comparative figures internationally?

SHEPPARD: The United Nations has them. A good source, by the way, for these kinds of comparisons is the Metropolitan Life Insurance Statistical Bulletin. Periodically they'll bring together a lot of statistical sources and do a lot of my work for me without my asking them. The National Center on Health Statistics may also have relevant data.

HENDRICKS: I wonder if you'd care to say anything about flex time (flexible working hours) in terms of employed males and working wives. It started in Germany because of traffic problems, not because of human beings.

SHEPPARD: Whatever the reasons, we're getting these changes. I don't know any studies and I don't want to speculate on what difference it makes for men as opposed to women, but the greatest appeal has been for women because they have all these home chores. I also didn't get into the whole emerging field of research on life management problems and how the job impedes the achievement of those life management tasks, especially for women.

HENDRICKS: The reason I asked the question is from going through the big Salase book, *Twelve Nation Time Budget Studies*. Those men that they could identify as following flex time patterns, the women in those same places had less free time allocated than did the men, while the reverse was the case when men were working constant hours. The flex time of the men was coming at the expense of their wives. I would assume that household obligations for women increase as men are underfoot more.

SHEPPARD: I have heard of some Swedish studies that disappointed the Swedish policymakers. Men take out of that freer time under flex time to maybe go hunting or bum around with buddies. They haven't changed the sex roles much at all, although one of the original purposes was to make it possible for the man to help the wife more and to be a father more. Cultural roles are very hard to change.

CAIN: I see a fork in the road for the gerontological movement more generally. There are some ironies here. At the very time at which liberal attorneys and others are campaigning for "down with mandatory retirement," on the basis of liberating a person to make a choice, that is being followed by the Senate and the House raising retirement to age 70. The question is whether there will be a follow-up point, hinted at in Juanita King's statement that we will up the age of eligibility to begin full pension, full social security. So we are working within the notion that it is a privilege to continue to work while your demographic data suggest that it is a necessity for survival of a society with any economic accountability. I see a classic warfare situation shaping up. It may be that a certain segment of the population is in jobs where there can be some flexibility or there can be a mid-career change, where there is intrinsic value in the intellectual work, professional work, or so forth, but at the same time it is apparent there is a lot of work that is a drag. Automobile workers by 55 are ready to get out of that place. How are we simultaneously going to meet both the freedom to continue to work and the demand-to-work issue on the one hand, and that's a contradiction, and meet the pleas of the policeman and the fireman and coal miner and automobile worker on the other, to get out of the labor force earlier? I see the gerontological movement wavering. I saw the National Council on Aging coming out of the Harris poll leaping from cultivating the image of the older person as exhausted, poor, lonely, ill-health, etc., to the image of the red hot mamas and papas now. Who are going to be the spokesmen for the old people who are left behind and are exhausted and frustrated with work?

SHEPPARD: You have seven questions there. Some of it, I

think shows some contradictions, but I'm not sure that all of it does, as you imply. I try to answer the questions in terms of allowing people an option to retire if they are in lousy jobs, and with somewhat decent income, while not forcing retirement on those who want to work and can work. Incidentally, the numbers that have been estimated that would continue to work after the age of 65 in the whole United States is at most 200,000. I don't understand why the opponents of the change are so emotional about it. It is reminiscent of the early days to get civil rights legislation, that all these millions of blacks would be coming in and all these women would be coming in and we can't have all those people. I think that the real segment we have to be concerned about are the very old population, like 80 and over, and they incidentally, are increasing at the greatest rate. Between now and the year 2000, the 80 + population will have increased by something like 130% in size whereas the young-old, 65-69, go up like 25%. I start out with a value position here. I want to make sure that the people in their 80's will be taken care of damned well. They're very expensive to take care of. If that's the case, it means that some of these young-old have to be kept in the work force to provide those transfer payments to pay for the decent care of the very old population. And I'm really talking about a dimension we have not discussed at all — the fantastic heterogeneity of that so-called older population, the 65 + population. Just with reference to age itself it is ridiculous these days to talk about "the" 65 + population. It is horribly heterogeneous and we must sooner than later start providing statistics, the government has to, and in our own research, with clear-cut purpose of using 65-69 and 70-74, and I'll settle now for 75 +. Fifteen years from now we're going to have to have 75-79 and 80 and over and so on. An 85 year old has little in common with a 65 year old, but we put them all together.

BEATTIE: If most of us look at the public policy debate on raising mandatory retirement five years, we're still staying with a constant of mandatory retirement. We really have not developed the kind of assessment capacities that we do when we hire people at any other age for a job and apply it throughout the lifespan. We're trying, societally, to stay off the hook. At the same time we're debating mandatory retirement and even the social security payment issues on the young versus the old. In the *New York Times* there have been editorials positing it as if the old are taking jobs from the young. Yet I hear what you've been saying, that many men are not really in the labor force at many points in their life span. I don't see the future any rosier, with our present underemployment and the black young and others without jobs. Their old age in the future is going to be very bleak. A big issue is the meaning, uses and allocation of the time over the lifespan, and the reward systems for that. It seems to me that part of this discussion is this question, not just of retirement or labor force, but of how we allocate time, its meaning and its uses. And that has to be built into a policy analysis. This five years to me does not say very much about the future. If we have longevity increasing, the issue is not going to solve itself very well, as you point out. The 85 and older group really are the pressure points of the future.

SHEPPARD: Last week I was at a meeting where a famous researcher kept using the 50 + population as the old group. He decided, because it's administratively convenient in his research, to use 50 + as a definition of old, and I took him to task for that twice in the last eight years. The first time he said to me, "When you get to be 50, you'll know, you'll feel old, Harold." But it bothers me. Policy-makers can be influenced by statistical reports and if they are going to look at data based on under 50 and over 50 to make policy, that is ridiculous, but so is it ridiculous to use 65 and over, and under 65.

CAIN: Two points. First, we should be reminded that the division between adulthood and old age, at least in law, is very recent. Blackstone's commentaries in England make no appreciable reference to anything but adulthood. A couple of years ago I was briefly with the Federal Council on the Aging, working toward a policy proposal for the frail elderly, and the definition of when frailty set in came up. I tried to compartmentalize, to make a three-tiered rather than a one-tiered view of old age and came up with the phrases "frisky," "frail" and "fragile." I took this out on the circuit and I was upstaged. Somebody said, "You're not a poet at all. The poet has already said, there are three stages in old age: the go-goes, the slow-goes and the no-goes." I took this to West Virginia and I came up with still a variation. At first you're frisky, then you're risky, and after that there's still corn whiskey. The other comment I want to make concerns your note about the heterogeneity of people past 65. It's becoming more and more apparent that counting forward from birth is no longer, if it ever was, any viable basis for determination of status in old age. I've been working (in wierd ways) on the proposal to count backwards from projected death. The demographic and statistical mentality would say you can't do that, especially on an individual basis, and the psychology says it would so upset people you can't do it. The fact is that in law at the present time, in administrative law and in court decisions increasingly, this is precisely what we are beginning to do: IRS, in dealing with the taxes on annuities; settlements dealing with industrial accidents of a worker at age 40 or 30 or 25; the amount a widow gets in settlement; the efforts of the black caucus and other minority caucuses to trigger eligibility to old age benefits at an earlier age because of a life expectancy. There are lots and lots of activities going, at least in the court, that suggest that we are slowly, but maybe surely, dealing with the heterogeneity issue.

SHEPPARD: In connection with the black aged, the Caucus for the Black Aged is slow because the statistical reality has now surpassed them. A black male, if he reaches 65, has the same life expectancy as a white male at 65. The argument that they ought to get their benefits earlier because they're not going to live so long is largely washed out. By the time a black woman gets to be 75 she's going to out live all the other people who are 75. There's a Darwinian principle here. If you are capable of getting to 75 and you're black, you've really got to be tough.

Chapter **4** THE FRICTION OF TIME
Access And Delay In The Context
Of Medical Care
Barry Schwartz, Ph.D.
University of Georgia

Time is scarce; it must be spent in the pursuit of collective
and personal goals with an economizing attitude. Thus conceived, the waste of time through waiting and delay must be socially as well as personally consequential. During the past few
years, I have had the opportunity to develop my interest in the
social costs of time waste by an analysis of data from a nationwide survey on utilization of health care services. Although I
will review here what I have learned from this inquiry (part of
which is reported in detail elsewhere [Schwartz, 1978a; 1978b]),
my main objective is to develop further its theoretical significance and to trace out some of its broader social implications.
My specific purpose is twofold: (1) to describe the consequences
of the time costs of medical care and to show how these costs are
reduced or inflated by the social context in which they are in-
curred, and (2) to demonstrate how the sources of time costs are
related to different aspects of this same structure. I will make
only one assumption about the point of view of the client. I will
assume that waiting is usually a negative or costly experience because it involves the foregoing of attractive alternative activities. However, what I am about to say raises the question of
whether this subjective point of view can be discussed apart
from the objective conditions to which it gives expression.

75

OBSTACLES TO THE UTILIZATION
OF MEDICAL CARE: MONEY
RATIONING VS. TIME RATIONING

Waiting time is experienced within the context of a social structure; waiting is also *used* by that structure for its own convenience. Thus, one may entertain two models of the distribution of medical and other kinds of services. In the first, which can be defined as the "normal exchange" model, medical care is provided exclusively on the basis of ability to pay. In the second, the "welfare" model, service is allocated according to need. One important respect by which these "delivery systems" are distinguished is the mechanism which brings supply and demand into a workable equilibrium. In the first model, the rationing criterion is money. In the second model, the rationing criterion is time; that is to say, a welfare system inundated by demand will apportion scarce services by the assignment of priorities. The rule of "first come, first served," or "service in order of urgency," or some combination of the two, thus replaces ability to pay as a method of allocation. One may express this synchronic relationship in diachronic terms: the more the costs of service become spread throughout a system and its accessibility equalized, the more dramatically time comes into play as a rationing criterion.

What seems to best characterize the contemporary order of medical care, at the national level, is a mixed system in which fee for service, fee according to ability to pay, and free service are combined. One is correct in assuming that within such a system the affluent use the more expensive services with short waiting times; the least affluent use less expensive services with longer waiting times. However, this does not mean that medical care among the more well-to-do is rationed by money alone. The situation is more complicated than that. Given a rather constant *rate* of supply of medical service, but a growing affluence and enhanced ability to afford it, even the fee-for-service establishment, because of increased demand,[1] is very often forced to resort to time rationing. A combination of rationing criteria may therefore be imposed by a single service unit. The richer a society becomes, then, the more it is forced to rely upon a method of rationing previously reserved for the poor. Two opposite conditions thus lead to the same form of allocation: time is used to ration service when *no one* can afford to pay and when *everyone* can afford to pay.

In short, the increasing importance of time in the distribution of medical care is brought about not only by a redistribution of service in favor of the poor but also by the general growth in society's affluence. These two distinct trends find convergent expression in both increased waiting time[2] and in the nearly unexceptional consistency with which waiting time is found to be a source of deep dissatisfaction with medical services.[3] Too much money chasing too few goods and services, thus produces inflation in the temporal as well as the monetary realm.

In this part of my paper, I want to summarize some findings on (1) the deterrent effect of waiting time on the utilization of medical service; (2) the separate effects on utilization of time and money costs and (3) the conditions under which it is possible for delay to inhibit utilization in the first place. What gives these findings their significance is the broader issue of whether we are presently living in a society in which money remains the major device for the effective apportionment of resources in general or whether time has begun to replace money as the *principal* restraint on consumption.

This same issue is raised by Daniel Bell in his treatment of "The End of Scarcity" in *The Coming of Post-Industrial Society* (1974: 456-475). Bell argues that as material shortage is overcome and the basic amenities come within the grasp of everyone, qualitatively new scarcities emerge and take on greater salience than they previously had. These scarcities relate to (1) information, (2) coordination, and (3) time. I will be concerned with the relationship between the latter two dimensions.

SOCIAL STRUCTURE AND TIME SCARCITY.

My guiding assumption is that the "opportunity costs" of time are most likely to be consciously reckoned in social systems which rely upon a high degree of coordination for the achievement of their goals, that is to say, where schedules, deadlines, appointments, and timetables are essential to the orderly conduct of everyday life. The modern metropolis is undoubtedly the most elaborate manifestation of this social form. In Hawley's (1950:309) words:

> The rhythmic functioning of the dependent [metropolitan] community, with its multiplicity of differentiated parts and its rapid tempo, requires a closely articulated timing system. Even such a minor thing as the failure of the milkman or postman to call at his regular time creates disturbances which may disrupt the activities in a number of interrelated units. Any interruption in the schedule of a transportation facility, any change in opening or closing hours of banks, stores, theaters, and other agencies is always productive of more or less confusion.

Simmel (1950: 412-13) expresses himself in this same regard:

> The relationships and affairs of the typical metropolitan usually are so varied and complex that without the strictest punctuality in promises and services the whole structure would break down into an enextricable chaos. Above all, this necessity is brought about by the aggregation of so many people with such differentiated interests, who must integrate their relations and activities into a highly complex organism. If all clocks and watches in Berlin would suddenly go wrong in different ways, even if only by one hour, all economic life and communication of the city would be disrupted for a long time. In addition an apparently mere external factor: long distances would make all waiting and broken appointments result in an ill-afforded waste of time. . . Punctuality, calculability, exactness are forced upon life by the complexity and extension of metropolitan existence.

These remarks, though made in specific reference to the city (*die Grosstadt*), also bear on communities which are functionally connected with and directly dependent upon the city.

Hence the importance of time and timing to the suburban way of life. In the words of Seeley, Sims and Loosely (1956: 64-65):

In Crestwood Heights time seems almost the paramount dimension of existence, not ony in the simple sense that all human events occur in sequence, and therefore in time, but rather because of the pervasiveness of time as a force in life and career patterns. There are constant demands for efficient work (that is to say, for the most economical use of time), for punctuality, for regularity, which call for an acute sense of timing. These are important factors in the estimation of success or failure.

An urban population with its ramifying interdependencies is almost compelled to adopt synchronized schedules. . . .The children have their school — which demands punctuality — scheduled appointments with dentists and dancing teacher, and numerous social activities. Home life is indeed often hectic. . . .But the very nature of secondary group life beyond the primary, family circle can hardly permit too much simplicity, and the resultant schedules are so demanding that the parents feel themselves constantly impelled to inculcate the virtues of punctuality and regularity in themselves and the child. . . .The activity promoted by [institutions] is regulated by the clock, and the schedule of one institution, unless it is definitely raiding the time and clientele of the other, must be fitted to the schedule of others within an inevitable tight competition for time. . . .The phenomenon which the Crestwooder calls "pressure" is caused by this concentration of demands into limited units of time.

Implicit in these statements is the assumption that small towns and rural areas, built as they are on a more limited, less differentiated scale, admit of looser schedules and more tolerant limits on synchronization. These systems are less "time dependent" (Schwartz, 1978c). That the pace and tempo of the city is faster and more hectic is a notion which, although deeply rooted in contemporary thought, has never been put to the test.

Of course, much is known of the extraordinary flexibility of "time sets" in traditional societies and of the resulting indifference of their members toward broken appointments, tardiness, and being kept waiting (Hall, 1959: 128-145); however, we know much less about time orientations among the diverse segments of advanced industrial orders. The scraps of evidence available seem to suggest that while small town and city residents are equally conscious of time, as measured by the accuracy of estimates of time of day (Lowin, cited in Doob, 1971: 82), city residents are more pressed for time, as measured by pedestrian walking speeds (Bernstein, cited in Milgram, 1973: 17).[4] The harried tempo of the city is also reflected in speeds, acceleration patterns and latency of traffic signal response of automobiles (Milgram, 1973: 17).

If the metropolis admits of less tolerant time-orientation than do smaller, less extensive networks of communities, and if delays are more likely to inhibit utilization of services among individuals whose activities are woven into the most closely synchronized systems, then the relationship between waiting time and service utilization should be most pronounced in metropolitan areas.

I tried to test this assumption by drawing on data from the project which I mentioned earlier. This nationwide survey was part of a comprehensive 1970 investigation of health care use, expenditures, attitudes and practices (Aday and Andersen, 1975). The information was collected by the National Opinion Research Corporation according to the general design of the Center for Health Administration Studies of the University of Chicago. Included in this survey are 3,210 heads of household who have a regular source of medical care and who reside in metropolitan areas, small cities, and rural towns and farms. In this survey, utilization of medical service was indexed by the number of office visits made by the respondent during 1970. Excluded from this measure are visits related to pregnancy and childbirth. The measure itself was obtained by an estimating procedure which combined information provided by the respondent, his doctor, or both.

The theoretically most important determinant of utilization is medical need. Because need is also significantly correlated with income and temporal access to doctors, I tried to take its effects into account. Assuming a person's health to be the best index of his medical requirements, I tapped four of its dimensions, namely, disability days, frequency of selected symptoms, days in hospital and self-reported health in 1970.

The office waiting time measure embodies an answer to the question "How long do you usually have to wait to see the doctor, once you get to his office?"[5] The ease with which a person can afford the monetary cost of care is indexed by total family income from all sources during the year 1970.[6]

I estimated the relative effects of health, income, and office waiting time on consumption of medical service by multiple regression. As I anticipated, need for medical service turned out to be the most important determinant of visits to a doctor's office. I also found that income has only a slight facilitating effect on office visits: the beta value is an insignificant .03. The corresponding beta for the office waiting time measure was − .05. This last outcome is significant (with appropriate controls)[7] well beyond the .05 level.

It is true that the effect of waiting time is very weak. In fact, I found that if the mean delay were increased by 30 minutes, the typical individual would make only .14 fewer visits per year.[8] By the same calculation, an increase of 15 minutes would produce .07 fewer visits. Such an effect is not a very substantial one. However, the purpose of my inquiry is not to predict *individual* behavior but to assess the *aggregate* effects of an increment in aggregated time costs. In this connection, small effects (like small increases in the rate of unemployment) may reflect massive consequences. Thus, a 15 minute increase in waiting time among the heads of the nation's 63 million households would entail a reduction of .07 × 63,000,000, or about four and a half million, visits a year. This includes only household heads. The reduction in office visits would be far greater if the same effect could be applied across the entire population.

The most relevant finding, however, was that visits to doctors seem to be inhibited by waiting time in metropolitan areas alone. In cities and suburbs, the effects of delay, as measured by beta coefficients, took on significant values of −.09 and −.10 respectively. (These are to be compared with income betas of .07 and .03). In non-metropolitan urban areas, rural towns and farms waiting time effects were insignificant. These findings conform to the assumption that delay is most consequential in highly differentiated and time-dependent systems. They also suggest that the influence of time costs relative to money costs is greatest in the same context. This configuration of outcomes cannot be due to the different characteristics of metropolitan and non-metropolitan people. After all, the city and suburb exhibit almost identical waiting time effects, yet differ grossly as to the makeup of their populations.[9]

The findings which I have reported are neither dramatic nor conclusive; however, they are at least consistent with the theoretical assumptions introduced earlier. As such, these findings admit of a number of questions and a number of tentative conclusions.

IMPLICATIONS

The first thing we must recognize is that the ultimate limit on consumption is the time expenditure it requires. As Linder (1970: 125) puts it:

> Even if our needs are infinite and production techniques continue to improve, there is a. . . possibility of the scope of continued consumption increases becoming exhausted. A time allocation analysis shows this indeed to be the case. The limit need not be set by our resources on the production side or by needs on the consumption side. The decisive factor can instead be a resource on the consumption side, namely, time. . . [I]f the supply of time is limited, and if time is a necessary resource, not only in production but also in consumption, then time will function as a restriction. The degree of utilization of consumption goods declines.

The facts which I have presented suggest that we qualify this statement. They show that, in relation to medical care, the inhibiting effect of time on consumption is limited to time-dependent metropolitan communities. However, the findings also suggest that, within these systems, delay is at least as formidable a barrier to utilization of service as is money. On the other hand, neither barrier seems to be consequential for individuals; only when their effects are aggregated do we sit up and take notice. Accordingly, the time barrier to medical care represents a social but not always a personal problem. Its ultimate effect is therefore to be measured in the sphere of *public* health.

Of course, even the social significance of these results may be negated by the fact that they relate to only one type of service, namely, medical care rendered by a regular or family physician. The popular notion is that the demand for this kind of care is highly flexible, that family doctors more often than not find themselves treating minor symptoms which do not actually require their intervention. And if busy people are deterred from consulting a doctor because of an uncertain delay, then the problem which they would otherwise bring to him could not be a very serious one. But the available evidence suggests this to be untrue. For example, Aday and Andersen (1975: 87-91) recently provided a group of 40 University of Chicago physicians with a list of 20 symptoms and asked them to indicate, in reference to each symptom and among five age groups, the percentage of patients who probably should consult a doctor. The percentage of respondents who actually did consult a doctor for symptoms experienced during the year was then compared with the physicians' ratings. The result showed that the respondents did not visit doctors more often than they should have (Andersen and Aday, 1975: 44-51). The manner in which the present discussion may be generalized is informed by this finding.

Regardless of the pressure of his personal commitments, and no matter how time-dependent the community in which an individual may reside, he will doubtlessly find himself indifferent to the time costs of many benefits. Inelastic demand is primarily responsible for this indifference. On the other hand, there are many goods and services whose consumption, by reason of very flexible demand and low money prices, is highly sensitive to the time it takes to procure them. Of course, it is not yet possible to say precisely how specific benefits order themselves along this continuum. However, it would seem reasonable to assume that if imperative medical needs may go partially unmet because of unacceptable time costs, then less pressing needs must be even more likely to be thus inhibited.

Regardless of the nature of goods or services, however, questions about the time it takes to procure them are most likely to be asked in contexts where time is scarce. In these settings, the familiar question "How much?" is most likely to be accompanied by another question: "How long?" Because the utilization of medical service is so heavily determined by need, it does not provide the most dramatic demonstration of this tendency. On the other hand, while the magnitude of the waiting time effect is relatively weak, its *pattern* justifies the theoretical statements which initially captured my attention. These statements embody the conviction that time and its waste can only be properly understood in the context of definite forms of social organization. The remainder of my paper is informed by this same conviction.

SOURCES OF DELAY

I have so far confined myself to the consequences of delay; I have said nothing about its sources. This is the problem I would now like to take up.

The "Service System" Model of Waiting Time

Up until very recently, academic interest in waiting time was limited to the realms of mathematical statistics and operations research. The volume and scope of application of work in these areas has grown phenomenally since Erlang's pioneering efforts during the first decade of this century (Morse, 1967). Application to problems in medical service delivery, for example, is now especially common. However, this kind of approach admits of intrinsic limitations.

Notwithstanding the many technical subtleties involved,

the basic idea of mathematical "waiting line" or "queuing theory" is a simple one. From any "service system", like a bank teller's counter, supermarket, or doctor's office, four dimensions are abstracted: (1) the volume and distribution of arrivals during a certain time interval; (2) the volume and distribution of service outputs during this same interval; (3) an operating rule or queue discipline, e.g., service in order of arrival or urgency, and (4) a service structure, e.g., single queue-single server, single queue-multiple servers. Given values and/or specifications for each of these four dimensions, it is possible to estimate the probabilities associated with different queue lengths and client waiting times as well as server idle times. It is equally possible to determine the arrangements which will produce specified waiting and idle times. The accuracy of estimates arrived at in this way depends of course on the validity of the assumptions upon which the computational model rests. Some of these have to do with the relationship between the length of a queue and the willingness of a client to join and stay in it and the speed with which that client is processed. There are may points at which these assumptions can depart from reality (Lee, 1966). However, the main conceptual problem inheres in the premises which are taken for granted. These are transparent enough: Queuing theory finds the causes of delay and congestion to reside at the same level of analysis on which they are observed. Only one assumption is advanced concerning the relationship between properties of the service system and the properties of the broader setting in which the system is embedded. The latter are held to be conditions which do not vary, constants within which input-output relations transpire. This assumption is of course untenable.

Classical queuing theory is at once too abstract and too concrete. It is too abstract in its exclusive preoccupation with the most general properties of service systems, that is, the volume and organization of arrivals and service. It is too concrete in that it operates exclusively at the miscroscopic level by focusing, in its application, on a particular service setting. By failing to distinguish between "endogenous" processes indigenous to that setting and the "exogenous" or macroscopic conditions which stimulate and inhibit them, queuing theory ignores the causes to which the dynamics occurring within the setting itself relate.

To say this is to make an observation, not a critical judgment; for mathematical queuing theory is no more than a way of resolving the common dilemma of whether to create formally sophisticated models of some process by over-simplifying certain features of the "sub-system" and ignoring the world beyond it, or to attend to the ultimate determinants of sub-system process at the expense of theoretical elegance. There is no need to deny the advantages and immediate utility of the first strategy to affirm the existence of questions which it leaves unanswered and the ultimate disadvantages of relying upon it exclusively.

In contrast to formal mathematical analysis, the sociology of congestion and delay involves the application of diverse perspectives, variables, explanatory and interpretive modes to those service system dimensions which are most relevant to the processing of clientele. Two basic foci are involved. The first concerns the way activities of service systems are structured into statuses, roles, authority and power relations, and how they are governed by moral rules and enforcements. These questions have been dealt with elsewhere (Schwartz, 1975: 63-131). This section of the present paper speaks to a second concern: the relationship between micro-and macro-system processes. The point of view which is brought to this concern holds service system parameters to be *intervening variables* which mediate between delay and the broader institutional factors which are its ultimate determinants.

EXCHANGE THEORY AND ECOLOGICAL APPROACHES TO WAITING TIME

From what can be presently determined, only one inquiry has ever approached the question of how service systems and social institutions are linked together in the determination of waiting time. This is a paper, written a few years ago, titled "Waiting, Exchange and Power: The Distribution of Time in Social Systems" (Schwartz, 1975: 13-46). The general assumption of this essay, which seeks to extend sociology's longstanding interest in social and economic inequality, is that an individual's access to service is determined by his location on the vertical dimension of society; its specific proposition is that the distribution of temporal access coincides with the distribution of power. This was found to be true in two senses: first, because a server's power is indexed by the scarcity of his skills and resources, those who desire his benefits generally cannot gain immediate access to him but must instead wait until others are accommodated; second, because the expenditure of time entails costs in terms of more profitable activities foregone, resourceful clients tend to make use of those servers who impose the least delay. This is to say that the powerful seek out the faster service they can afford, and that those who would serve them must compete by minimizing their waiting time. By contrast, people who are unable to pay, or cannot pay full price for the service they receive, may avoid delay only if they are willing to settle for no service at all. Hence the tendency for the more affluent to obtain medical care from private doctors; the poor, from clinics, where they are kept waiting. However, the substitution of money for time is possible only to the extent that faster alternative services are available to those who want them. When there are few or no alternatives, as when a service is monopolized, servers have no incentive to compete for the good will and patronage of clients by increasing the volume of service or, in some other manner, reducing client delay. Class differences then become attenuated and everyone faces long delays. The assumption that waiting time is affected by both income and opportunities is to be referred to as the "resource - availability theory," as it was originally designated.

What I want to do now is to assess the validity of this argument and to try to deepen our understanding of the linkage between individual delay, the makeup of medical service systems and the organization of the society in which these systems are located.

The main supposition of the resource-availability theory of access and delay is that waiting time for medical and other ser-

vices is longest for society's least resourceful groups. This supposition is borne out in the NORC sample. The average high income head of household in that sample is delayed for about 39
minutes in the waiting room of his regular doctor before being
seen by him. The mean for the low income head of household is
64 minutes.[10]

Now if delay in the acquisition of service were mainly
determined by money, then waiting time differences among
sub-groups would be explained by their income differences.
That is to say, waiting time variation along the horizontal
dimension of social status would be accounted for by the differential positioning of status groups on the vertical dimension of
economic power. The facts, however, are inconsistent with this
assumption.

In our society, race is the politically salient dimension of
status. I found that it is also an important correlate of waiting
time. High income blacks wait 59 minutes — 21 minutes longer
than high income whites. Low income blacks wait an average of
93 minutes, which is 37 minutes longer than whites of comparable income. The findings are inconsistent with a perspective
which asserts that time and money are the only elements to be
combined in the procurement of service. Although I called upon
a number of arguments to explain the findings, none succeeded.
Similar regional patterns and the absence of differentials in appointment waiting time seem to rule out discrimination as an explanation of the observed racial inequalities. I also entertained
an argument that race and income differences in delay would
vanish if the length of waiting time were weighted by its value.
This, of course, can only mean that time is least precious among
poor people and blacks. Because this assumption touches upon
the subjective meaning of time and time waste, I might enlarge
upon its rationale.

I have suggested that the distress of waiting is a manifestation of the opportunity costs of time, that is to say, the value
foregone in waiting that could have been put to use elsewhere.
Economists, of course, assert that the value of foregone time is
directly proportional to earned income (see, for example,
Becker, 1965; Nicholas, et al., 1971). It is the poor, therefore,

who are said to be least likely to "balk" or refuse to enter a queue; they are also assumed least likely to "renege" or abandon a queue after having joined it. While the poor may have something *else* to do besides sitting and waiting, they might not have anything *better* to do. This kind of argument, which sounds reasonable enough, is not only advanced in theoretical discussion; it is also put to use by econometricians in their estimates of the value of time.

If earned income is to be used as a measure of its worth, then black time must surely be considered less valuable than white time. However, there is another reason to attribute inferior value to the time of black people. This is based on a cultural rather than an economic premise. Because of a reputedly slow-paced and easy-going life style, blacks are assumed to be insensitive to the demands and strictures of time. In contrast, whites consider themselves to be more respectful of schedules and appointments, and more willing to gear their fast-paced lives to the clock. This difference is expressed in the image of the harried but punctual white bureaucrat, on the one hand, and the black "Step 'n Fetch It" caricature, on the other. It is also expressed in the notion that "White People's Time" is qualitatively different from "Colored People's Time"[11] It would be reasonable to assume, then, that while blacks wait longer, a longer wait is not as meaningful to them as a shorter one is to whites.

These ideas can be readily tested if we are willing to make one assumption, namely, that those whose time is most scarce and valuable are those who feel most oppressed when it is wasted. Of this sense, expressions of impatience provide at least a crude measure. Such an indicator, which orders respondents according to their "satisfaction with waiting time in doctors' offices and clinics" was obtained from an attitude and opinions segment of the NORC household survey.

I find that when waiting time is held constant, this measure of impatience is independent of income; however, it is significantly associated with race, with blacks exhibiting the least tolerance of delay. This difference is most pronounced among low income heads of household where, regardless of the length of delay, the percentage impatient among blacks exceeds the percentage among whites by at least 10 points.

These findings mean that there really is a difference between "White People's Time" and "Colored People's Time"; however, its direction contradicts popular assumption. It is the black, not the white, who feels most oppressed by delays. Accordingly, if the magnitudes of white and black waiting times were weighted by their "unit costs," measured in terms of expressed dissatisfaction, the white-black inequality would be considerably larger, not smaller, than it now appears.

I tried in other ways to discount the effects I had observed, but to no avail. For example, since blacks and poor people tend to be disportionately represented in medical facilities which have relatively long waiting times, that is, clinics as opposed to private physicians' practices, and in walk-in as opposed to pre-arranged appointment systems,[12] I thought race and income differences in waiting time might vanish if source of care and appointment status were simultaneously controlled. In fact, they were reduced by an average of less than five minutes.

By confining my attention to the differential recruitment of white and black, wealthy and poor, into various kinds of service systems, I neglected the way these facilities are spatially distributed in relation to the people who use them. The importance of this relation resides in the localized congestion and time costs it is capable of generating. Of course, medical facilities and their clients are distributed *within* as well as *among* communities. I considered each distribution in turn, taking note first of the significant between-community variation.

I began by classifying all respondents according to their place of residence, and comparing average waiting times. I discovered, however, that while high income people and whites are overrepresented in communities which display the shortest waiting times (suburbs, non-metropolitan cities and rural towns as opposed to metropolitan cities and farms), income and race differences in waiting are reduced by no more than a few minutes even when residence and the physician-population ratio are controlled together.

If the unequal apportionment of medical facilities *among* communities fails to account for inequalities in client waiting time, is there any reason to assume that unequal apportionment of care *within* communities would be a more useful source of information? That turned out to be a pivotal question, for the more I thought about it, the more transparent the problem became and the more unavoidable its attending explanation. The reason is as follows.

In any community or metropolitan area, medical services tend to follow wealth: the densest sector of their geographical concentration is centered in regions of affluence (see, for example, Dorsey, 1969; Dewey, 1973; Navarro, 1974). For example, the present survey shows that travel time to regular source of care is inversely proportional to income. However, this survey also shows that travel time is *directly* proportional to office waiting time. The farther from a medical service concentration a person may reside, then, the poorer he tends to be -- and the more competition he faces from others similarly located when he seeks out medical care. This is because individuals, regardless of their income, tend to select those physicians whose offices are closest to their homes. Affluent people, therefore, not only travel shorter distances to their regular source of care; they also have more doctors to choose from; the poor, on the other hand, spend more time traveling and have fewer choices. In a community with one or more concentrations of medical establishments providing regular care for their clients, competition among *physicians* will be most intense at the center of these concentrations; client waiting time will be correspondingly minimized. However, competition among *clients* will be most intense at the periphery, and waiting time will be maximized.

The principal reasons why blacks wait longer than whites of comparable income relate directly to what has just been said. Because of a long established tradition of residential segregation, along with the general poverty of the Negro population, high and middle income blacks are now more likely to reside in low income communities than high and middle income whites. Conversely, low income whites are more likely than their black counterparts to reside in affluent communities, especially suburbs. This is why blacks in the survey sample are more likely than whites of comparable income to be walk-in patients and to utilize clinics. But there is another factor operating. Because the members of the medical profession are overwhelmingly white, they tend to live among and practice upon white patients. Although doctors are among the first to abandon an area when its income diminishes (Dewey, 1973), there are always a few remaining to serve the nearby white poor. Regardless of their size and income, then, there are likely to be more physicians in white communities than in black communities.

Because there are comparatively few offices and clinics to meet the demands of the black and the poor, those which are available tend to be inundated. Accordingly, what is important as far as waiting time is concerned is not so much the assortment of income and race among diverse sources of care as the distribution across space of the least advantaged parts of the population, on the one hand, and the medical establishment, on the other. Waiting time is in this sense a phenomenon of human ecology as well as individual preferences for time costs as opposed to money costs (as is suggested by many economists) and the internal efficiency of doctors' offices and clinics (as is suggested by modern queuing theory).

Indeed, it is not so much that the black and the poor visit slower facilities; rather, the facilities are slower *because* they serve the economically and socially disadvantaged -- because they are inundated with people having literally nowhere else to go. It is for this reason that income and race effects are maintained when source of care is held constant.

I tried to verify this conclusion by going back to the original questionnaires and selecting out from the total sample those respondents in the Chicago area for whom office waiting time and address of physician could be ascertained. My objective was to determine how well class and race effects on waiting time hold up when local differences in the availability of doctors is taken into account. If these effects are mainly the result of prevailing patterns of segregation, then they should be substantially reduced if we hold the ecological factor constant by focusing in on narrow segments of the metropolis. But the 127 cases were simply spread too thinly throughout Chicago's 75 communities and suburbs to allow for this kind of analysis. It was therefore necessary to aggregate the data into zones and sectors with the help of secondary documentation.[13]

I discovered that as one moves from the inner city through the outer city to the suburbs, the number of physicians per 1000 population increases from 75 through 87 to 94. Mean waiting time decreases from 95 through 65 to 27 minutes. (The Loop, which is only represented by three cases, is excluded.) However, it was not possible to do comparable internal analyses of each of these three zones. Residential segregation is pronounced enough in this metropolis to make for a sample in which 46 percent of the whites obtain their care, and no doubt reside, in the suburbs (home addresses were destroyed to preserve confidentiality); 98 percent of all blacks reside and visit doctors in the city. Therefore, no area-specific black-white comparisons could be made. And, in the suburbs, no class comparisons are possible: all suburban respondents were classified at the high-income level.

Although the data showed that significant income differences in waiting time persist in both the inner and outer city, these differences almost vanished when source of care or travel time (an index of local availability of doctors) was held constant. Income effects also persisted in the two sectors of Chicago which contain most of the sample (the southern sector, where the doctor-population ratio is .66 and the mean waiting time is 93 minutes, and the western sector, where the doctor-population ratio is .48 and the mean waiting time is 100 minutes). But, for the most part, these effects are also explained by source of care and travel time.

These findings are based on too few observations to warrant any hard and fast conclusions. Moreover, they do not *fully* account for the relationship between income-level and waiting time. On the other hand, the direction of the results is consistent with the argument for whose sake they are presented. They show that while income effects on waiting time persist when city-wide variation in physician availability is reduced by dividing a city into zones and sectors, almost all of these effects are explained by source of care and local levels of availability. As the geographical unit of analysis becomes smaller, then, waiting time differentials attributable to income are radically attenuated. Taking these already unstable differences, and projecting them down to the separate local communities of which the larger zones and sectors are composed, we are led -- inevitably, it would seem -- to anticipate their total disappearance.

What all this adds up to is not only a demonstration of the shortcomings of our previous understanding of "waiting, exchange and power" but also a documentation of an alternative point of view which takes us beyond it. This alternative is embodied in the perspective of "temporal ecology," which concerns the way time and its investment is affected by disjunctures in the spatial distribution of social groups and the institutions which serve them. Such a perspective informs the resource -availability theory by showing *how* resources and availability are joined together in the determination of delay. The resourceful, we find, do wait less, but not only because they deliberately substitute money for time. We also find that providers of a service in ample supply do indeed maintain shorter queues, but not only because they consciously strive to do so. Whatever the individual motivations involved, delay will be inversely proportional to resources because of the way resourceful and resourceless people are spatially organized.

IMPLICATIONS

The total time cost that our society incurs in obtaining medical care is substantial. In addition to the time it took to get to a doctor's office in 1970, I found that, on the average, a household head spent 45 minutes waiting once he got there. Since in that same year there were about 63 million heads of household in the United States, and because each of them made approximately four visits to his regular source of care (Aday and Andersen, 1974:36), the total waiting time expended comes out to over 189 million hours, or about an eight hour work day for almost 24 million people. Of course, this figure does not take into account waiting times for those without a regular source of care, nor does it include waiting times of spouses and dependents. It ignores delay at offices to which patients are referred by their regular doctor. Moreover, it assumes that all patients make their doctor visits individually; in fact, many are accompained by others who wait with them. This is especially true, of course, where children are concerned. The total time cost involved in obtaining medical care is therefore many times greater than that estimated for the particular subjects of this investigation. The total cost would be even more dramatic if it were aggregated across all retail and service sectors.

Now what I have tried to do in this second part of the paper is to get at the factors which determine the way these time costs are spread throughout the social structure. I began my inquiry by considering a simple exchange model of access and delay. That model has one basic assumption: that time is freely substitutable for money. The higher the income, therefore, the stronger the tendency to carry out the substitution. Given the choice between a private physician who charges per visit 15 dollars plus 15 minutes of waiting time and a clinic which charges three dollars plus three hours of waiting time, the affluent patient will pay the 15 dollars in order to save almost three hours of valuable time; the least affluent will prefer to spend three hours of relatively worthless time in order to save money.

This arrangement, it would seem, allows patients to utilize a service with that particular time-money price combination which is cheapest for them. For the poor, high time cost and low money cost is best; for the affluent the optimum combination is a low time cost and a high money cost. What we have, then, is a theoretically neat and equitable system. However, as soon as we take this system to be a description of reality, we come up against a number of contradictions. We find that blacks substitute time for money more readily than whites, regardless of their income or source of care. Furthermore, the relationship between income and waiting time is for the most part independent of the type of facility a group chooses to frequent. The poor, like the blacks, wait longer at private offices as well as clinics.

The problem with a simple exchange model, I found, is

that it assumes a measure of choice which is really not there for all clients to exploit. That is to say, the time price an individual pays for medical care depends not only on the way he chooses to allocate his income but also on something which has nothing manifestly to do with time or money, namely, the location within the broader metropolitan context of the local community in which he resides. The connection between these seemingly independent factors is brought about by the spatial distribution of physicians. Income is a predictor of waiting time because medical care concentrations are centered in the most affluent sectors of a community where doctors are most plentiful in relation to the number of nearby clients. By contrast, high income people who reside in low income communities lack the opportunity to substitute money for time, for their choice of care is limited to the periphery of service concentrations where competition is most pronounced.

Because blacks are most likely to fall into this latter category, their waiting time exceeds that of whites who are similar to them in other respects. Racial discrimination in the administration of medical care therefore need not be assumed to account for the race differences we have observed. On the contrary, race is related to waiting time by the same ecological principle which links income to waiting. Independent race and income effects exist because residential segregation by income and race are independently superimposed upon one another.

The present findings thus relate the well known spatial dimensions of the local community to its less visible temporal dimension; they enable us to see for the first time, and with some degree of precision, how the ecological concentration of service units affects the time costs and time budgets of their clientele. The main question, however, is one of generalizeability: whether we must assume that space-time linkages relate exclusively to health care or whether they apply as well to the distribution of other goods and services. If, as the evidence suggests (Dewey, 1973: 117, 129), the location of medical facilities is affected by the same factors as those determining the location of service units in general, then we must assume that the socially disadvantaged incur greater time costs in all aspects of their consumption. This means that the thesis of "The Poor Pay More" (Caplovitz, 1963) must be applicable to time as well as money. This is so not because of the consumption habits of the poor or the selling practices of the marketplaces which serve them; what matters is the spatial distribution of these market-places. That is to say, the reluctance of most providers to locate in poor communities makes for greater competition among resident consumers and longer queues at existing establishments.

The facts that I have summarized demand that mathematical and economic models of delay and time waste be located within the broader context of social organization. For in the medical context, at least, delay is no more than one expression of an overarching macroscopic linkage between class, status, and space. Specifically, the distribution of waiting time is an organic phenomenon of the way class and statuses are ecologically sorted with respect to the institutions which serve them. Time deficits are generated, accumulated and organized by the laws of *spatial* segregation.

CONCLUSIONS

In bringing this chapter to a close, I wish to devote my attention to the more general implications of what I have learned about delay in the context of medical service. As I try to condense and tie together my materials, I may therefore take the liberty of turning from a serious to a more lighthearted example.

In my initial statements, I suggested that as a society grows more affluent, money becomes less effective as a rationing device. Time cost takes its place. It occurs to me that the carnival is a microcosm of this arrangement. I am not thinking about all carnivals; only those in which payment of a gate fee provides free access to all rides and amusements. What is important, however, is that these benefits are not absolutely free.

Any experienced patron knows that they are dearly paid for by time spent in line. This same patron also knows that the more popular the amusement is, the longer the line will be. As a result, a person may have to resign himself to the less enjoyable sites if he is to have any fun. Once the initial fee is paid, then, choices are made within the constraints of a pure time economy; here, the queue replaces money as a pricing mechanism.

My discussion of waiting time as an obstacle to the use of medical service may be subsumed under this carnival model, provided it is modified to take context into account. If our carnival is located in a time-dependent environment, like the complex post-industrial metropolis, the behavior of its "previously committed" or harried patrons will be most sensitive to the time price embodied in the queue. If the carnival is situated within a loosely coordinated environment which is less dominated by the schedules and deadlines which make for time scarcity or "overload," then patrons will be relatively insensitive to the queue's time price. On the other hand, given the volume of demand on each carnival amusement, along with the speed and efficiency with which each processes its customers, this analogy breaks down when called upon to depict the ultimate sources of waiting time. This is because the carnival's fit with the *social organization* of the metropolitan community is not as snug as its fit with that community's typical method of *allocation*. Specifically, patrons of the carnival do not reproduce their environments by spatially segregating themselves according to achievement and color. As a result, these patrons cannot be differentially sorted among carnival amusements as they are among services in the real world.

The ecological aspect of patterned inequality in access to service not only points to what is wrong with looking at life as a carnival; it also shows what is theoretically at stake in this paper. That implication has directly to do with the concept of social distance. The conclusions I have already drawn suggest that we might profit by decomposing this concept into its various dimensions.

Commonly, three types of social distance are distinguished: (1) vertical distance, which is dealt with by the students of social stratification; (2) horizontal distance, which is the concern of ethnic and race relations; and (3) spatial distance, the subject of human ecology. Much writing in sociology and many debates relating to social policy have to do with the way these dimensions are connected to one another. I have introduced an additional dimension, temporal distance, and have tried to show how it relates to these older, classical concerns.

I consider the temporal dimension to be important because all social activities, from the cultivation of intimate relationships to the consumption or utilization of goods and services, require and may therefore be inhibited by the expenditure of time. This expenditure may be broken down into three components, namely, the amount of time it takes for one peson to reach another with whom he desires or needs to interact (which might entail a trip to another part of a building, street, or town), and the amount of time a person must wait for another's presence once he has made himself available for interaction. Obviously, time in interaction can be spent only after these two initial barriers are overcome. Return trips, delays encountered in the process of traveling, interruption and delay after an engagement is underway, and so forth, are simply variations on this basic three-part division of time investment.

Although students of human ecology routinely deal with time, they have confined themselves to only one component of temporal distance, namely, the time required to move from one point in space to another (part 1 of my trichotomy). This emphasis is reflected in Hawley's (1950: 288) formulation:

> Space and time are separable from one another only in abstraction....Space is experienced within the framework of a time system. Space has been described as a time-cost variable. The distance that may be traveled for any purpose, assuming a given amount of time at the disposal of the traveler, is contingent on the speed and efficiency of existing transport facilities. Hence the territorial scope of the community and, to a large extent, the number of individuals who live in close mutual dependence, are fixed by the time required for the overcoming of distance. Similarly, the distribution of units within the community varies with the time used in movement. A temporal pattern is implicit in each and every spatial pattern

In this "dyadic" model, temporal distance (given a certain level of transport technology) is simply a function of the separation of two different points in space. So long as we focus only on one component of temporal distance, the relationship is no more complex than this. However, in order to fully understand the ecology of time, we need to account for the temporal distance which separates two people located at the *same* point in space. This is of course a problem which concerns the second component of temporal distance: waiting time. The solution of this problem requires the substitution of a distributional model for the dyadic one, that is to say, a model which directs our attention to the differential array in space of a number of stationary points (providers of service) and a number of mobile and mutually competing points (clients). This model, as I have tried to show, is capable of accounting for time costs attributable to delay as well as locomotion. In doing so, the model not only gauges the friction of space in terms of time; it also relates the friction of time to the distribution of people over space.

Vertical, horizontal, spatial, and temporal distance are highly integrated in our society. Knowledge of an individual's location along the vertical dimension implies, in a probabilistic way, his location on the horizontal, spatial, and temporal planes. Any movement along one dimension is typically accompanied by a displacement along other non-ascriptive dimensions. Thus, upward mobility often involves the kind of residential change which brings about an improvement in temporal access to certain sources of goods and services. Caution is needed, however, when it comes to the problem of describing the nature of this relationship. Melbin (1977:1) expresses what is probably the most widely held point of view by arguing that "human events occur within four-dimensional boundaries, in a space-time container.... There is no pure spatial or temporal ecology. Only space-time ecology." This statement, which makes explicit what is implicit in Hawley's point of view, does not seem to me to be adequate in an analytic sense. By failing to distinguish between the functionally dominant and subordiante aspects of the "spacetime container," Melbin leaves us with the impression that time and space are merely two sides of the same coin. This cannot be. There is an inherent asymmetry in the relationship. Temporal distance and costs are unquestionably the consequences, not the causes, of spatial distributions. Of course, ecological patterns themselves only give expression to exigencies of other orders, namely, status differentiation (which is sustained by circumscription of social contact) and class differentiation (which is predicated upon money and what it can buy [Weber, 1948]). The integration of vertical, horizontal, spatial, and temporal distance is therefore hierarchical in character. Time distance is created by the spatial expressions of status boundaries, whose specific coordinates are ultimately related to the market position which defines the vertical dimension of class.

Access to medical and other services cannot be understood independently of these hierarchically patterned distances. In a metropolitan society of rising affluence, where there is a growing awareness of the basic needs of all citizens, access to service is increasingly determined by ecological patterns. A man's position in the marketplace of the emerging time economy is affected in a significant way by his location on its territorial dimension. Accordingly, if the utilization of an important service is inhibited by the time needed to acquire it, that inhibition must be traced beyond the organizational confusion and inefficiency of service facilities, along with the often sluggish indifference of their personnel, to the macroscopic plane of social organization.

NOTES

[1]Perlman (1969: 108-111) shows that the number of physicians per 100,000 population, corrected for changes in age composition, was no higher in 1964 than in 1908. He also points out: "As wealthy individuals at any point in time use more physicians' services than do the poor (although probably not at a rate as high as their comparative wealth), our index simply suggests that we have fewer physicians relative to our wealth then we would have had in 1908."

[2]In their study of the effects of a compulsory, universal health insurance

plan (Medicare) in Montreal, Enterline and his associates (1973) find an 11 percent increase in office waiting time after the establishment of the plan. Thus, as
the costs of service are spread throughout a population, waiting time increases.
(No other similar longitudinal study of waiting time has been brought to my attention.)

[3]In a national sample (to be described above), dissatisfaction with office
waiting time is expressed by 35 percent of all heads of household. Only availability of night care and cost of care elicit higher levels of discontent. Comparable
levels of dissatisfaction are to be found in research by Hulka (1971), Alpert
(1970), and Deisher (1965).

[4]The absolute difference in walking speeds among pedestrians in a number
of large, moderate and small towns varies by less than 10 percent. However, this
effect, which is statistically significant, is as strong as one could expect, given the
difference between walking and running.

[5]The interview schedule breaks down responses to this question into seven
categories: (1) seen immediately; (2) less than 15 minutes; (3) 15 to 30 minutes;
(4) 30 minutes to 1 hour; (5) 1 to 2 hours; (6) 2 to 4 hours; (7) over four hours.
Persons falling into the second through the sixth intervals were assigned the
value (in minutes) of the interval midpoints. The category "seen immediately"
was assigned a value of 1 minute. The last open-ended category was assigned a
width of 3 hours (1 hour longer than the preceding interval and 2 hours longer
than the interval preceding that). The midpoint of this last interval, which contains 2 percent of the cases, is 5 and a half hours.

[6]This measure does not take into account the fact that some heads of
household obtain care at reduced fee or at no charge at all. But most of the physician fees covered by third parties are paid through voluntary insurance and include services related to hospitalization (Andersen, et al, 1973: 49; 53-54). There
is no comparable information in this regard as it relates to office visits in particular. Yet, while family income may not be the best measure of individual
vulnerability to medical costs, it is an excellent measure when applied to individuals aggregated into income groups. As Andersen and his colleagues (1973: 12)
have shown, outlay for personal health services as a percentage of family income
is about twice as high among the poor as among middle and high income groups.

[7]In this computation, the time it takes to obtain an appointment and travel
time between home and doctor's office are controlled. Although both variables
are negatively correlated with utilization, neither correlation is significant. I cannot say for sure why this is so. I suspect, however, that part of the reason is that
appointment waiting time and travel time are known quantities which can be incorporated into a predefined schedule, while office waiting time is typically an
unknown quantity for which time cannot be allocated.

[8]The unstandardized beta is .00474.

[9]Furthermore, a separate analysis showed that these outcomes are independent of income and race.

[10]The waiting time distribution is skewed in the direction of longer delays.
The median waiting time, therefore, is several minutes shorter than the mean

waiting time. This has no bearing on the present discussion. The analysis to be reported above was replicated with a waiting time measure dichotomized at 30 minutes. The same patterns emerged and identical conclusions were drawn.

[11] John Horton (1970: 44) advances the view that "Colored People's Time" is a variant of lower class "street time." However, he also points out that "middle class Negroes who must deal with the organization and coordination of activities in church and elsewhere will jokingly and critically refer to a lack of standard time sense when they say that Mr. Jones arrived 'CPT' (colored people's time)." It is Herskovits' (1941: 153) contention that colored people's time may be traced to the lax time sense of traditional African society.

[12] For full discussions of service scheduling and its relationship to waiting time, see Fetter and Thompson (1966) and Johnson and Rosenfeld (1968).

[13] Doctor-population ratios by community area were made available to me by Donald Dewey. The concentric and sectorial divisions of the city and associated doctor-population ratios are reported in his monograph (1973).

REFERENCES

Alpert, Joel J. *et al.* 1970. "Attitudes and Satisfactions of Low-Income Families Receiving Comprehensive Pediatric Care." *American Journal of Public Health* 60 (March): 499-506.

Andersen, Ronald, *et al.* 1973. *Expenditures for Personal Health Services: National Trends and Variations, 1953- 1970.* Washington, D.C.: Department of Health, Education, and Welfare.

Aday, LuAnn and Ronald Andersen. 1975. *Access to Medical Care.* Ann Arbor: Health Administration Press.

Becker, Gary. 1965. "A Theory of the Allocation of Time." *Economic Journal* 75 (September): 493-517.

Bell, Daniel. 1973. *The Coming of Post-Industrial Society.* New York: Basic Books, Inc.

Caplovitz, David. 1963. *The Poor Pay More.* Glencoe: The Free Press.

Deisher, Robert W., *et al.* 1965. "Mothers' Opinions of their Pediatric Care." *Pediatrics* (January): 82-89.

Dewey, Donald. 1973. *Where the Doctors Have Gone.* Chicago: Chicago Regional Hospital Study, Illinois Regional Medical Program.

Doob, Leonard W. 1971. *Patterning of Time.* New Haven: Yale University Press.

Dorsey, Joseph L. 1969. "Physician Distribution in Boston at Brookline, 1940-1961." *Medical Care* 7 (November-December): 429-40.

Enterline, Philip E., *et al.* 1973. "The Distribution of Medical Services Before and After 'Free' Medical Care — The Quebec Experience." *New England Journal of Medicine* 289 (November): 1174-1178.

Fetter, Robert B. and John D. Thompson. 1966. "Patients' Waiting Time and Doctors' Idle time in the Outpatient Setting." *Health Services Research* (Summer): 66-90.

Hall, Edward T. 1959. *The Silent Language.* Greenwich: Fawcett Publications, Inc.

Hawley, Amos, 1950. *Human Ecology.* New York: Ronald Press.

Herskovits, Melville. 1941. *The Myth of the Negro Past.* Boston: Beacon.

Horton, John. 1970. "Time and Cool People." Pp. 31-50 in *Soul,* edited by Lee Rainwater. Chicago: Aldine.

Hulka, Barbara S., *et al.* 1971. "Satisfaction with Medical Care in a Low Income Population." *Journal of Chronic Disease* 24 (November): 661-673.

Hurtado, Arnold V. *et al.* 1973. "Determinants of Medical Care Utilization: Failure to Keep Appointments." *Medical Care* 11 (May-June): 189-198.

Johnson, Walter J. and Leonard S. Rosenfeld. 1968. "Factors Affecting Waiting Time in Ambulatory Care Services." *Health Services Research* (Winter): 286-295.

Lee, Alec M. 1966. *Applied Queuing Theory.* London: Macmillan.

Linder, Staffan B. 1970. *The Harried Leisure Class.* New York: Columbia University Press.

Melbin, Murray. 1977. "Time Territoriality." Unpublished Manuscript.

Milgram, Stanley. 1973. "The Experience of Living in Cities." Pp. 1-22 in *Urbanman,* edited by John Helmer and Neil A. Eddington. New York: The Free Press.

Morse, Philip. 1967. "The Application of Queuing Theory in Operations Research." Introduction to *Queuing Theory,* edited by R. Cruon. New York: American Elsevier.

Navarro, Vincente. 1974. "A Critique of the Present and Proposed Strategies for Redistributing Resources in the Health Sector and a Discussion of Alternatives." *Medical Care* 12 (September): 721-42.

Nicholas, E., E. Smolensky and T.N. Tideman. 1971. "Discrimination by Waiting Time in Merit Goods." *American Economic Review* 61 (June): 312-323.

Perlman, Mark. 1969. "Rationing of Medical Resources: The Complexities of the Supply and Demand Problem." *The Sociological Review.* Monograph 14 (September): 105-119.

Schwartz, Barry. 1975. *Queuing and Waiting: Studies in the Social Organization of Access and Delay.* Chicago: University of Chicago Press.

Schwartz, Barry. 1978a "Time and Black People: A Study of Temporal Access to Medical Care." *Sociological Focus.*

Schwartz, Barry. 1978b "The Social Ecology of Time Barriers." *Social Forces.*

Schwartz, Barry. 1978c "Queues, Priorities, and Social Process." *Journal of Social Psychology.*

Seeley, John R., R.A. Sim, and E.W. Loosley. 1956. *Crestwood Heights.* New York: Basic Books.

Simmel, Georg. 1950. "The Metropolis and Mental Life." Pp. 409-424 in *The Sociology of Georg Simmel,* edited by Kurt H. Wolff. New York: The Free Press

Weber, Max. 1958. "Class, Status, Party." Pp. 180-195 in *From Max Weber,* edited by H.H. Gerth and C. Wright Mills. New York: Oxford University Press.

Weber, Max. 1964. *The Theory of Social and Economic Organization.* Glencoe: The Free Press.

COCHRANE: It seemed to me that it was not actual facts you were talking about; it was the economics of this particular problem prior to obtaining health care. How does time enter here? It seems perfectly obvious that rich people can do more or less what they please and poor people have to wait. What is the difference here between health and absolutely everything else? I mean what, in a sense, is different here for these individuals and any other kind of services? How can you make a special case for this?

SCHWARTZ: Time cost is what I'm trying to explain. Variation in time cost is what I'm trying to explain.

COCHRANE: No, no. You link those words, but they are not demonstrably linked. You link them by saying them, but they are not linked simply by you saying them.

SCHWARTZ: Waiting time involves cost because it entails a foregoing of alternative activities. It's in that particular sense that it involves a cost. One can also examine the cost of time in terms of irritation, impatience or in terms of income foregone as a result of travel and waiting time.

COCHRANE: It's the linkage between time and cost that I'm essentially questioning.

SCHWARTZ: All I can offer are two indexes of cost. One is obvious. Waiting time always involves a forfeiture of alternative activities, or alternative investments or commitments, however you want to describe them. That, after all, is true by definition. I provided a second indicator of cost: impatience. You say, "What does it have to do with health?" I tried to show that waiting time inhibits the frequency of visits to doctors' offices. I also indicated that impatience inhibits the frequency of visits to doctors' offices. I also tried to indicate an overall pattern of that inhibition. A third point that you introduced is that poor people obviously have to spend more time cooling their heels than affluent people. But it isn't at all obvious that regardless of income, Blacks have to spend more time waiting than whites. Why is that? The obvious response, or the response I've always gotten, is that Blacks, after all, have to go to clinics. But when we hold source of care constant we obtain exactly the same pattern. I think I've answered all of your questions.

GLASSNER: You said to him that it is somehow the forfeiture of alternative activities or frustration — what were you saying that that is?

SCHWARTZ: These are indicators of the cost of time.

GLASSNER: I guess that the only thing I can say is to read *Time and the Cool People* or Suttles' *Social Order of the Slum* to demonstrate that for many groups those have nothing to do with their reality. You take these surveys instead of going out and seeing what matters to these people.

SCHWARTZ: I'm quite puzzled by your response. What I've presented here are differences in time costs, or differences in waiting time. I said that I could have weighted each of these differences by a measure of impatience, which is one indicator of what's important to people.

GLASSNER: By whose standards?

SCHWARTZ: I think that it's really impossible to hold a dialogue. Now what you're holding fast to is a hard core symbolic interactionist position. That seems obvious to me. If you're going to say that all of this survey material is worthless, then I don't see how it's possible to have a discussion.

GLASSNER: Forget symbolic interactionist or the survey. My point is that for some people, for example some street corner persons, a primary activity that is highly valued is the forfeiture of other activities in favor of what you describe as waiting.

SCHWARTZ: Let's say that it takes eight hours to go someplace by car and that it takes half an hour to fly. What you're saying is that that difference is not important. I'm taking into account the way the difference in time is interpreted. I'm not sure I know quite how to respond to that position. This is what I tried to take into account by presenting the material on impatience. After I presented the material, I said that perhaps this pattern of waiting time difference would disappear altogether if we took interpretation of time into account. The only measure of interpretation that I had was the response which patients gave to the question, "How do you feel about the time you usually spend waiting in doctors' offices or in clinics." This is the only index I had. I tried to show the pattern of results obtained with that impatience measure would not alter, would not suppress, the differences that we observed. That measure would have had the opposite effect: it would have magnified them.

ZERUBAVEL: You're talking about time costs and money costs as two alternative costs. Are you also considering the symbolic difference between the two, or just a practical one?

SCHWARTZ: You're asking the same question — the symbolic difference. The ony measure that I have of that symbolic difference is the impatience index. That's the only one I have.

ZERUBAVEL: It has nothing to do with his talking about the meaning of the data. I have no problem with that, I am just asking about the distinction between money and time, the distribution of different symbolic significance of time and money.

SCHWARTZ: If you look at the literature in economics, for example, you find the assumption of an interchangeability of money and time. The assumption is that people are free to substitute one for the other. What I'm pointing out is that they aren't at all free, they are constrained by the ecological patterns that I've described.

HENDRICKS: But you're saying that the one is the reverse of the other, that if you consider time important, then money is less important. I think that's what people are getting upset about — that there's some sort of nicely, neatly balanced thing that says, "Oh, gee, whereas now we're getting more time conscious and money conscious, therefore these are things that are exchangeable." What they're saying is for different groups this may not operate the same way.

ZERUBAVEL: In the beginning you were talking about temporal distance, that if you use temporal distance you don't need a measure of spatial distance.

SCHWARTZ: No. This is Hawley's idea. There's a long discussion of the subject in Amos Hawley's *Human Ecology*. Now what I've tried to show here is that even when you "control" for space, that is to say, when you have a patient sit in the waiting room of a physician's office (in that sense you're "controlling" for space), ecology does have an effect on waiting time, but this effect doesn't have anything to do with the friction of space. Hawley was talking about travel time in his treatment of the friction of space. You don't have to talk about travel time to see how ecology effects time costs. That is, ecology effects time costs because of the differential distribution of institutions and people. This is what I tried to show but this is not the point that Hawley is making.

HALL: Two things that I don't know whether you've considered. They are on the problem of impatience. Is impatience itself something that you can measure in any objective way as you've tried to do or rather has to do with the subjective temporality of the person involved? In other words, I can be waiting for medical care in a number of different ways. One is to find a bureaucracy, a medical care service bureaucracy, an alienating experience. Alternatively, I can be a person who has a briefcase with me, has my work on my investment decisions to make and so forth. Also I'm wondering if impatience is not something that has to do with status differential. Perhaps low income people, low income Blacks, feel imposed upon in having to deal with this alien, highly rational system of medicine.

SCHWARTZ: Incidentally, there's a good deal of literature in psychiatry and psychology on boredom, on the consequence of fantasy on impatience, and so forth. These, I assume, all find expression in the impatience index that has been used in this investigation. Again, I would be happy to discuss these concerns with you in some other context. Unfortunately, all I have here is a handful of IBM cards and I'm drawing what conclusions I can from these cards. I hate to be put in a position where I have to defend survey research against other forms of research.

HALL: No, I'm just pointing out that we need to maintain a critical understanding of what impatience means.

SCHWARTZ: Sure, but we also have to understand what we're talking about in context of the data if the discussion is to have any point at all.

UNIDENTIFIED: I have a cleaning woman, who happens to be white rather than Black, who is constantly expecting people to be putting her down. She doesn't get along with doctors, she doesn't get along with hospitals, her son has had a horrible motorcycle accident and everything is irritating her about the whole thing. Is that part of your impatience?

SCHWARTZ: I can't account for where the respondent puts that pencil mark of his. I assume that the variation that we observe, because it's after all associated with values, gives expression to something complicated, subtle. . .

DAVIS: I've got a question about the ecological explanation. I find it to be, at least from my point of view, very compatible with the data as you presented it. But, like all explanations you can create explanations that are compatible but need not be true. How would you test the ecological explanation. The data, of course, don't do that.

SCHWARTZ: It's impossible to test it on the national sample. So what you have to do is to get data on the way physicians and patients are distributed over space within a particular city or a community. And then you have to somehow divide that town up into zones or sectors. If differences in waiting time are indeed generated by the differential distribution over space of people and the institutions which serve them, then, when we focus in on particular segments of the city, we would expect the pattern to disappear. This is to say, the associations should reduce to zero. And that is exactly what happened in the Chicago data. It's because the association between two variables disappears when I introduce this "test variable" that I feel content with the explanation that I gave.

HENDRICKS: What was the test variable that you used for the ecological test?

SCHWARTZ: Ecology itself. That is to say, I examined income differences in waiting time within particular zones and sectors of Chicago. In doing so, I reduced the variation in physicians per capita. When that variation is reduced, the income difference disappeared.

HENDRICKS: You had, then, that kind of specific data on individual respondents?

SCHWARTZ: Yes, I did.

HENDRICKS: Another question. What about the initiating complaint? If I go to a physician for a ruptured appendix, 15 minutes is going to be far more important than for a common cold.

SCHWARTZ: Oh yes. No, I did not have that information. Patients were asked how frequently they experienced certain symptoms over the year but they weren't asked what the problem was on a particular visit.

HENDRICKS: Don't you think that that would be an important criterion if you're going to determine the relevancy of time in a health care setting?

SCHWARTZ: It would be helpful to have that information.

HENDRICKS: Well, I think more than helpful.

SCHWARTZ: But I don't see how the absence of that information would cause me to alter the conclusions that I've drawn.

HENDRICKS: I don't think I could comfortably attribute the differences to what you're calling here ecological variables in the absence of some attitudinal variables.

SCHWARTZ: Again, I'm not sure what the structure or the logic of your argument would be. What is the alternative argument? Also, impatience is one index of attitude.

UNIDENTIFIED: It seems to me that nature of the complaint has some relationship to cost and impatience. For example, if you've got a ruptured appendix you're going to go to emergency; you're not going to sit in the doctor's office. If the nature of the complaint is severe enough, then it is worth your time in the doctor's office waiting for the doctor. You don't get impatient if you have to wait over something serious. You might get more attention if you have something serious or more impatient sitting and waiting on a routine matter. So it seems to me the nature of the complaint has to be investigated.

SCHWARTZ: When I was examining differences in impatience, I went into that. The self-reported health scale indicated how frequently respondents experience pain, and so forth. There's a group of other attitudinal measures. I wanted to see if the differences between Whites and Blacks would hold up if these attitudinal measures were held constant. They hold up. But the point that I'm trying to bring across here is that the impact of housing segregation goes far beyond the problem of schools, the problems of busing, the demoralization of ghetto existence. The kinds of spatial distributions that we've been talking about and the contradictions and tensions which emerge from housing segregation by income and race also extend to the province of time. What I'm trying to do is link up the relationship between time and space to the context of social organization. What I try to point out at the end of the discussion is that housing segregation generates (or probably generates) not only time cost in the medical sphere, but in all aspects of consumption, and in social relationships in general. This is the point I'm trying to elaborate on.

GLASSNER: Did you control for race of doctor?

SCHWARTZ: No.

UNIDENTIFIED: I wonder if, for my sake, you would reiterate one more time for the retardees the relationship between space and time cost.

SCHWARTZ: As I understand it, the common sense view is that poor people and Blacks have to spend more time in obtaining services because they obtain services at what might be called low-speed institutions, like clinics. This is the conventional view. Another view is that, in any case, these differences aren't important because poor people don't care how much time they wait. Black people don't care either. I tried to provide evidence which is inconsistent with that view. Also, I tried to show that the differences we've observed, and the differences you've referred to in your question, are produced or generated by a factor that has to do with human ecology: the disjuncture between the distribution of people over space and the distribution over space of the institutions which serve those people. Time costs, then, are generated by the principles of human ecology as opposed to factors of an organizational character — "the office is inefficient," "she isn't a very good receptionist," and so forth. These things are important, there's no question about that. What I've tried to do, however, is to highlight the importance of *ecology* and go beyond Hawley by showing that our understanding of the relationship between time and space isn't at all exhausted by arguments having to do with the "friction of space", that is, speed of transportation, and so forth.

Chapter 5

ABEYANCE PROCESS AND TIME: AN EXPLORATORY APPROACH TO AGE AND SOCIAL STRUCTURE

Ephraim H. Mizruchi, Ph.D.
Director, Maxwell Policy Center on Aging
Syracuse University

Few would deny that a fundamental problem in all societies, at some time in history, is the existence of surplus populations. A cursory reading of the historical literature on Western societies beginning, for example, with the decline of the Roman Empire will provide ample evidence that the phenomenon of too many people in society at a particular point in time was associated with dynamic processes of action and reaction, strain and conflict. Two dimensions of this phenomenon require articulation: the role of age cohorts and categories, and social control. The underlying structural processes and transformations can be approached by conceptualizing them in temporal terms.

As a preliminary assumption it is well to keep in mind that a population perceived as "surplus," either by participants in society or observers (e.g. historians), is not necessarily superfluous. Whereas a "surplus" population may be perceived as such only temporarily, a "superfluous" population is likely to be viewed as having neither a present nor a future place in a given society. A surplus population in American society today is clearly those youths and other age cohorts whom we may expect to finally integrate into the occupational structure. In marked contrast are the retired and elderly for whom the relatively near future holds only dependence and death. The elderly are more likely to be perceived as a superfluous, rather than surplus population. Thus the anticipated condition of a population in terms

112

of future states of society orients members of that society to the differential value of age cohorts.

It is in the nature of society, if Simmel was correct,[1] that as size of population increases so does impersonality. A corollary to this is that subjects become transformed, in our minds, into objects and, as such, they may be manipulated and constrained as societal requirements become manifest. The very terminology, "surplus population," implies people viewed *en masse,* people who must be dealt with in some way because there are too many of "them" to fit into the contemporaneous structure. They must be dealt with because as a mass which is less integrated into the social structure than others they are less subject to the surveillance and control of society. Social control, as Piven and Cloward have reminded us, is a concern when rapid change is present in society, and as time passes and control is assured, the so-called surplus population recedes from the societal consciousness.[2] But time-rate of absorption is an important determinant of the process of control and this requires that societies develop patterns and structures which assure that the outcome of asynchronization between surplus personnel and available positions does not threaten the existing order. It is to these patterns and structures that our attention is drawn.

Abeyance. The capacity of society to enhance or inhibit the absorption, integration and control of personnel is dependent on the relative effectiveness of what I call the abeyance process.[3] This process may be conceptualized as operative on the macro, micro and mediating levels of a society. Through institutions and organizations, groups and persons participate, knowingly and unknowingly.

Abeyance is a holding process. At the organizational level large masses of people may be "warehoused," to use a similar term, until status vacancies become available in other organizations. At the personal level impulses, motives and desires are postponed until both opportunity and normative justification allow goals to be attained. This process, viewed as the time-rate of absorption at the organizational level and the time-rate of personal attainment of goals at the individual level is essential to the effective functioning of society. Because it is essential, abeyance is typically associated with institutionalized patterns. How does the process work and what are some of the typical patterns associated with it historically and contemporaneously? Our effort, in this paper, will be brief.

The Beguines of Medieval Europe. An excellent example of abeyance may be derived from studying the emergence, the interaction and the decline of a women's movement in the Rhineland and the Low Countries of Western Europe during the Medieval period. The beguines were a lay order of women whose spiritual mission in life was, normatively, the pursuit of good works. They came into existence in the cities to which many unattached women had migrated from rural areas. Historians agree that in the urban context women, at least by the 13th century when the beguines became organized, constituted a surplus population. But the source of this surplus was not *simply* an imbalance of the sex-ratio at birth or the survival capacities of women. The surplus resulted in large part from a contraction of status positions and roles in the kinship structure. Because some men had begun to join monasteries, others were going off on crusades, others had gone off to war, and still others could not afford to take wives, the opportunity for a woman to assume a role in the kinship structure diminished. As unattached women they were perceived as a threat to the community. Initially these women organized to pursue the only tasks available to them: those which required limited training, aiding the sick and catering to the urban poor.

To legitimate their mission beguines, unacceptable to church authorities, justified their existence by espousing a religious orientation similar to the Brethren of the Free Spirit and other millenialists who rejected the right and necessity of the Church to mediate between the person and God. While varying conditions in the Church and the larger society influenced the extent to which they were viewed — at any point in time — as heretics, one thing is clear: The beguines developed an organized pattern of urban communes which absorbed, during the period between 1200 and 1600, large numbers of surplus women.

More significantly the beguines, unlike nuns — who take

vows for life — could leave the commune as other opportunities, i.e., status vacancies, emerged. Thus their relationship to the organization was intended to be temporary rather than permanent. When other opportunities, whether work or family, expanded, the beguines contracted. The organization held these women while other societal processes caught up, so to speak, with the imbalance.

As one of many types of organizations the beguines were unique because they absorbed surplus rather than superfluous populations. Because these unattached women could aspire, in time, to alternative opportunities and because they could demonstrate their value to community and society by their good works they were tolerated, then accepted. The heretic label was replaced, in at least one instance, by the appellation, "*Goode kinder vie men heet beginjes.*"[5] As an institutionalized pattern they helped cushion the impact associated with the time-lag in expansion and contraction of status vacancies in diverse organizational contexts.

The beguines provide but one example of the abeyance process. I have studied mandatory education, bohemianism, the Federal Writer's and Artists Projects of the WPA and still other patterns in an effort to articulate how societies deal with the time-lag of absorption of surplus populations. A number of organizational characteristics are associated with the rate of absorption of populations. Among these are: (1) inclusiveness-exclusiveness of membership criteria; (2) degree of integration of the organization; (3) degree of hierarchical relationships; (4) division of labor; (5) degree of commitment expected of members; and (6) the degree to which the activity is institutionalized within the host social structure. While time does not permit more than mere listing of these factors it is nevertheless important to note that temporality is associated with each one.

Ho 1: The more inclusive the membership the faster the rate of absorption, e.g., educational organizations;
Ho 2: The less the degree of internal integration, e.g., the Federal Writer's and Artists Projects, the faster the

rate of absorption;

Ho 3: The less the degree of hierarchical organization, e.g., bohemianism, the greater the rate of absorption;[6]

Ho 4: Over-commitment to an organization, as in the case of Greedy Institutions (Coser), inhibits the rate of contraction;

Ho 5: The more institutionalized the pattern, e.g., education, the greater the motivation to participate in structures which hold population in abeyance.

These are but a few examples, suggestive of the dimensions which can enhance our understanding of how time-lags at the level of social structure are cushioned by organizational patterns. That people in organizations are more under control while those who are unattached are less controlled - and thus vulnerable to participation in rebellious activity - requires little comment.

Transitional Status. Within an organization there are structures which hold *individuals* in abeyance as well. Glaser and Straus,[7] for example, have suggested the concept "transitional status" which denotes

> ...time in terms of the social structure. It is a social system's tactic for keeping a person in passage between two statuses for a period of time. He is put in a transitional status, or sequence of them that determines the period of time that he will be in a status passage. Thus the transitional status of the initiate will, in a particular case, carry with it the given amount of time it will take to make a non-member a member - a civilian is made a soldier by spending a given number of weeks as a basic trainee; an adolescent spends a number of years 'in training' to be an adult. (p. 85)

Using the Army as an example suggests still another form of internal abeyance. The many technical training schools in the

United States Army Air Corps during World War II, were manpower pools which held combat soldiers in abeyance until they were needed in battle, as during the mass evacuation of many troops from these schools during the Battle of the Bulge in 1944 and 1945. This helps explain why daily physical training and continuous upgrading and reinforcement of combat skills was an integral part of the soldier's activities while attending school. Indeed, as our study of mandatory education suggests, what goes on in school generally is clearly not as important to a community or society so long as young people are held in abeyance in relation to the labor market and, simultaneously, under control. The values placed on education and the legal sanctions which reinforce attendance make education one of the most effective abeyance structures in American society.

Socialization and Patterning. In order for abeyance processes to work it is necessary first to socialize persons in ways which enhance these processes and to reinforce the socialization process with group and organizational activities. The most general and useful descriptive concept with respect to socialization for abeyance is the Deferred Gratification Pattern, originally formulated by Schneider and Lysgaard.[8] While the DGP was most closely associated, in the sociological literature, with variations by social class, there is ample observation of ethnic patterns which suggests that other variables are similarly associated. Not only do people in the middle classes in the United States tend to control their impulses to a greater extent than those in the working and lower classes with respect to sex, spending, and aggression but, according to my hypotheses, they are better at waiting in all contexts and at anticipating future conditioning, (*c.f., e.g.,* in this context Schwartz'[9] work on waiting and queuing.) With the help of a whole array of values and norms like, "keep at it, success is just around the corner," Americans are taught to hold *themselves* in abeyance.[10] When asynchronization in the system occurs, these patterns play a role in the capacity of persons to cope with the holding process. Religious explanations, for example, including notions about life after death, tend to reinforce patterns of deferring gratification among some segments of the population of elderly in Judeo-

Christian societies. Sometimes, under extreme conditions, the holding pattern fails or another - like the beguines - is too late in emerging and a higher probability of rebellious collective action results. At still other times, as with the Calvinist experience, a rigorous system emerges which controls time and abeyance in an extremely effective manner. All of these examples attest to our assumption that societies do not allow for the random expression of impulse and that the patterns which exert control enhance the abeyance process.

However, since socialization alone is incapable of controlling behavior it is necessary to explore the organizational patterns which reinforce the DGP. Our quotation from Glaser and Straus suggests statuses and roles which reinforce holding patterns. It is safe to hold that all interaction involves impulse control, but engagement in organizational activities which include complementarity and reciprocity, coordination and integration, yields greater increments of reinforcement than do informal social interaction as size and complexity of organization or group increases tend to enhance awareness of one's need to be patient, that in time one will be able to pursue desirable goals. For these patterns to effectively reinforce there must be supports in the larger social structure. In a relatively complex society there may be pressures exerted which inhibit the process.

Timing, Spacing and Status Vacancies. It is important to keep in mind that a substantial portion of societal members consciously and intentionally behave in ways which enhance the cushioning of asychronization between status vacancies and personnel. A substantial body of literature based on demographic and survey research has been accumulating for at least 20 years on timing of pregnancy and child spacing.[11] This should come as no surprise to the social scientist since one of the most conspicuous variable social patterns in American society is the delay of marriage by relatively higher class persons. But the motivation, and thus the constancy and predictability of the pattern, is probably explained not only by the structuring of life styles - including greater concern and opportunity for extended educational and career involvement - but also by personal motives. Relative affluence allows for greater opportunity to "sow one's wild oats," to take time to decide what to do with one's life. It is sufficient to remind ourselves, in this context, that normative, cognitive and idiosyncratic factors must be explored in order to explain the connections between personal behavior, group expectations and societal synchronization and asynchronization.

We are not suggesting, in this context, that there is a necessary correlation between apparent societal needs and the behavior of persons and groups. The structuring of behavior in a society may create strains in the system which contribute to severe imbalances between personnel and status vacancies. The classic study of Irish countrymen, as Arensberg and Kimball[12] called them, in which it was observed that the unwillingness of the aging father to relinquish control and ownership of his farm to his son until quite late in life led to relatively late marriages between persons whose fertility levels were in decline. The result was a low reproduction rate which, from some points of view, limited personnel for status vacancies in the agricultural sphere. It is well to note that from still another value perspective, that of stability, there were no strains. One more example, related to cognitive motivation, suggests how asynchronization may emerge out of reproductive patterns. During the early part of the 19th century in England, when the factory system was expanding, it was economically feasible to have many children. The more children working, the greater the income for the family as a whole. As factory methods changed and fewer workers, i.e., children, were employable a surplus population emerged. Without work and without school, children roamed the street panhandling and committing diverse crimes. Engels,[13] in his study of the British working class, provides a description of the scene much like one would derive from a reading of Dickens. This particular imbalance was directly responsible, as Musgrove[14] shows, for the rise of mandatory education and child labor laws.

Time, Age and Social Policy. Our foregoing discussion demonstrates that the acute or relatively chronic problems associated with surplus populations in society can be better understood if we become sensitized to abeyance at the macrosocial, microsocial and mediating levels of conceptualized social systems. One of the major contributions of social science research to the formulation of social policy is to articulate how already ongoing processes provide enhancement or inhibition of emerging societal problems. The best way to do this, we believe, is by expanding basic knowledge and concepts as we focus on both perceptible and imperceptible sources of these problems.

The abeyance concept sensitizes us to the role of social structure and other forms of social patterning in the process of adaptation, maladaptation and change on the personal and group level to dynamic conditions which typically emerge out of largely unplanned but often predictable phenomena in society. Focusing on abeyance helps us see that formal occupational positions are not the only status vacancies which make a difference in society. The traditional view that jobs alone will provide a solution to the problem of surplus personnel appears myopic when we employ a wider lens through which to view social structure. Historical data and sociological insight, when joined, can contribute to an awareness of alternative sources of status vacancies.

Our distinction between surplus and superfluous populations, we feel, is critical to understanding the complexity of the problems affecting diverse age cohorts. To date the kinds of structures which are designed to absorb the elderly are more appropriately referred to as *terminal* rather than *abeyance* structures. While this distinction will require considerably more thought and exploratory observation it is immediately clear that the relationship between these two types of structures and the host communities and society are different. Similarly, the kinds of internal organization of these structures, their formal and informal goals, and the consequences of their activities will be different in significant ways.[15] At this juncture it is sufficient to note that policies dealing with the cohort of elderly should be directed to transforming *terminal* structures into *abeyance* structures, to changing superfluous populations into surplus populations, in anticipation of reintegration into status vacancies which provide meaningful, challenging and productive activity. Raising the level of awareness of policy makers to these patterns represents our initial effort.

FOOTNOTES

1. See the author's, "Urbanism, Romanticism and Small Town in Mass Society" in Paul Meadows and Ephraim H. Mizruchi; eds. *Urbanism, Urbanization and Change,* Reading, Mass: Addison-Wesley, 1969. Revised, Second Edition, 1976. I thank Mark Mizruchi for suggestions regarding this particular issue.
2. F.F. Piven and R. Cloward, *Regulating The Poor,* New York: Random House, 1972.
3. My first explicit usage of the term "abeyance" appears in "Bohemianism, Deviant Behavior and Social Structure," paper read at the Annual Meeting of the *Society for the Study of Social Problems,* San Francisco, 1969. The idea appears in some of my earlier work. CF. e.g., *Success and Opportunity:* A Study of Anomie, New York: The Free Press, 1964. p. 75.
4. *CF.,* in this context, a recent book by Robert Lerner, *The Heresy of the Free Spirit in the Middle Ages,* Berkeley: U. of California Press, 1972. More complete documentation, based on other sources will be presented in a book which I am currently writing. My treatment of these issues is included in E. Mizruchi, "Alienation, Mediating Processes and Social Control," *8th World Congress of Sociology,* Toronto, 1974; "Social Structure, Social Integration and Abeyance," *American Sociological Association,* Annual Meetings, Montreal, 1974; and "On the Uses of History in the Development of Social Problems Theory," Annual Meetings *Society for the Study of Social Problems,* New York City, 1976.
5. The Flemish is translated, "Good children who are called beguines." (My translation) In this context see, E. W. McDonnell, *The Beguines and Beghards in Medieval Culture,* New York: Octagon Books, 1969; and D. Phillips, *The Beguines of Medieval Strasbourg,* Stanford: Stanford U. Press, 1941.
6. L. Coser, *Greedy Institutions,* New York: The Free Press, 1974.
7. B. Glaser and A. Straus, *Discovery of Grounded Theory,* Chicago: Aldine, 1967.
8. L. Schneider and S. Lysgaard, "The Deferred Gratification Pattern," *American Sociological Review,* 18 (1953), pp. 142-9.
9. B. Schwartz, *Queuing and Waiting: Studies in the Social Organization of Access and Delay.* Chicago: University of Chicago Press, 1975.
10 Mizruchi, 1964.
11. Recent examples of this type of research are, "R.M. Stolzenberg and L. Waite, "Age Fertility Expectations and Plans for Employment," American Sociological Review, 42 (1977), pp. 769-781; H.B. Presser, "The Timing of the First Birth, Female Roles and Black Fertility," *Milbank Memorial Fund Quarterly.* 69 (1971), pp. 329-361; H.B. Presser,

"Perfect Fertility Control: Consequences For Women and the Family," in C.F. Westoff, et al. (eds.), *Toward the End of Growth: Population in America,* Englewood Cliffs, N.J.: Prentice-Hall, 1973, pp. 133-144.

12.   C. Arensberg and S.T. Kimball, *The Irish Countryman.* New York: Harcourt, Brace, Jovanovich, 1937.

13.   F. Engels, *The Condition of the Working Class in England,* Trans. and Ed. by W. O. Henderson and W. H. Chaloner, New York: Macmillan, 1958. This book first appeared in German in 1845.

14.   F. Musgrove, *Youth and the Social Order,* Bloomington: Indiana U. Press, 1964.

15.   Two important dimensions which we hope to explore, are the varying orientations to and consciousness of time in these contexts. An example of one type of study dealing with these dimensions is R.G. Kuhlen and R. H. Monge, "Correlates of Estimated Rate of Time Passage in the Adult Years," *Journal of Gerontology.* 23 (1968), pp. 427-433.

ZERUBAVEL: I was particularly impressed in the beginning by what you mentioned about impersonalization. I think that it can be seen as one major historical variable that influences the differences in the conception of what is old age. The theme is excellent to explain how old age is seen. The problem is impersonalized on a societal level.

MIZRUCHI: Peter Laslett's work on family structure before the industrial revolution suggests that certain kinds of changes which we assume in social relationships, assumptions about integration of the elderly into kinship structures and the like, probably do not correspond to the reality of the situation. Since starting to think about Laslett's work, and now having looked at more and more historical material in the last four or five years, I've become very cautious about attributions of taken-for-granted conceptions of large structural changes.

ZERUBAVEL: The focus of the problem of old age was in the family, right?

MIZRUCHI: That's an assumption that's made. The evidence shows that the elderly were in two-person families in Western preindustrial society, except where they held the wealth and power into old age. Under those circumstances their children lived with them. This is quite a different conception from the idea that the nuclear family is an emergence of the industrial revolution.

ZERUBAVEL: Is there any evidence that in premodern times aging was considered a societal problem?

MIZRUCHI: No. If one looks at legislation with respect to these matters, one finds all kinds of dirty dealings with large masses of people, including the elderly. For example, the Enclosure Acts were designed in part to force people off the land, so they would have to go to cities and work in factories--they needed factory labor--which created other kinds of problems, including squalor and tuberculosis.

LOPATA: Just one question on information that's not in your paper. Where did Engels talk about these issues?

MIZRUCHI: That's in his book, *The Condition of the Working Class in England.*

CAIN: Thanks for the abeyance concept. I've been circling around the periphery of this for a long time. You were talking about something related to one of my first efforts at grading essay exams, teaching from Robert Barry's *Social Disorganization* back in the late 1940's and early 1950's, and there had been a discussion of the one boy going off to study engineering, another going on to be a priest, and so forth. A student in the exam said, "The boys all left for the city and therefore the girls had a social change." Also, dealing with the so-called hippie movement, I was reminded of a little trick I pulled on the class a few years ago. I walked in one day and said, "Imagine ourselves being up here someplace godly, looking down on American society, and we want to maintain order. Over a long time we've had about two or two and a half million people coming into the labor force every year and wanting housing and marriage and all those things. All of a sudden we have about four million people knocking on the door every year. What do we do?" And then I said, "Well, start stringing them out on drugs, promote homosexuality, stash away a dozen people in a pad, get out in tents and communes. All of those radical break-aways from the conservative society."

GLASSNER: Did you ever hear Dick Gregory's speeches on that? When he was touring campuses at that point, he said, "I want you all to go back to your surburban communities and pick up on all that dope they're putting in there. Maybe they'll stop shifting it into the ghetto. Now they have to take care of you for awhile, because there are too many of you guys."

CAIN: I was struck also by the notion of rites of passage and the absence thereof in our society. In the Introduction to *Rites of Passage,* there was the comment that maybe part of the problem in American society is that we have no longer the bunched up rites of passage, the coactivity. In our society we've tended to substitute legal age for rites of passage, so every individual, on becoming 16, goes down to the driver's license place, and on becoming 21 goes down and gets his I.D. and goes out and gets drunk. The twist is that abeyance is seen as negative. To be held in abeyance would be seen as depriving or denying. It may be that our going to individual legal age for status transition, instead of bunching up and having ceremonies, is the negative for the purpose of identity, for the purpose of celebrating of the life course transition.

LOPATA: What you're saying is that it fragments the person.

CAIN: Yes, the freedom of individuality, instead of being a blessing, turns out to be negative, in that we don't have a peer group, we have ourselves. We got the driver's license, we registered for the draft.

MIZRUCHI: From the point of view of self-actualization, we transform ourselves. From that point of view of course it's negative because, as I suggested earlier, abeyance involves a transformation of subjects into objects.

MONGE: A case that I think illustrates a positive aspect of abeyance structure is the modern beguine, the Peace Corps. One other thing on abeyance structures and where they might go awry. Is it the case that the beguines and similar kinds of things were caused by an abeyance structure gone wild, that is, too many people went into monastaries, too many men went off to war, to the Crusades?

MIZRUCHI: There's very little literature on beguines. That's one of the interesting things about this area. There are probably about a dozen pieces of serious scholarly work in this area, and I have had to go beyond this into the German literature of the Marxists, because they're the only ones dealing with abeyance, from the point of view of women's rebellion movements. What

I'm really saying is that it is not sufficient to think of surplus populations as a result of demographic or biological forces, as is traditionally the case, but that one should see this as a result of institutional processes, organizational processes. Things go on in society, society is constantly changing. Obviously my conception here is somewhat cyclical. The existence of the elderly as a surplus or superfluous population can be conceptualized as something wrong with our institutional system, that there are not structures, again getting back to the rites of passage that Dr. Cain is talking about, what Schneider called deficiency theory. There is a deficiency in the social structure; the system is incomplete in that it does not respond to the needs and desires of large masses of people. We have a one-track mind. We value work so highly in Western Society that any solution has to be in terms of formal conceptions of work when, at the same time, we realize that a substantial amount of the work that we do is characterized by boredom, by alienated work. Again I don't want to overly romanticize because our data on assembly line activity do not simply support the 1844 Marx, the romantic Marx.

MONGE: What I'm getting at, is that abeyance structures like the Crusades, which I think were a matter of deliberate policy, or the Peace Corps, which is a matter of deliberate policy, or the Social Security system of 1935, again a deliberate policy -- are all things that went wild. Another example is educational systems. I heard on the radio the other evening that by 1985 we will have 10 million college graduates, of which 2.7 million will not find "appropriate jobs." What I'm saying is that we have abeyance structures set up as a matter of deliberate policy, with forethought, and they have gone wild. Where's the corrective?

MIZRUCHI: Again, Rolf, we have a problem here of a value position. Why has it gone wild? It's only gone wild if we think of advanced education in instrumental terms. But advanced education as end value, as a value in and of itself, intrinsic and so on could not hurt the society. So we have 15 million extra people drumming around who could pick up a book and enjoy themselves with it. It can't hurt us.

LOPATA: It was only about twenty years ago that persons still had to write that women in the modern world should be educated. They argued to educate women in colleges because, after all, they're going to be raising sons who will hold jobs. The ideology that education is only for appropriate jobs I think is part of that tremendous pushing in American society for occupation, which has made life miserable for many women and has made the isolated household, the hanging loose, and so forth. It has been a really wierd emphasis in American society: that set of values above all other values--friendship, extended family, all kinds of relations--are put back for the man's occupational career.

GLASSNER: It strikes me as interesting that we have reversed what a famous Greek philosopher proposed: that what we call liberal arts education be reserved for those who would never work in our sense of work. And now you've got to have it and it's for work.

FRASER: There is, indeed, a demand that education be used for furthering the individual's aims, "go back son and make more money" and all that. But there is wisdom in many members of our society. Among the people we know, our children's age, I could name a dozen who by studying and then doing something else are closer than their elders to the classic Greek idea of education for the sake of its beauty rather than its usefulness. Our son-in-law went to college, read his Dante and is remarkably happy making custom built furniture. He finds nothing wrong with it. Problems like the linear demand of education tend to be taken care of by the people who are involved. I think that's great.

MIZRUCHI: I can't help but respond to your comment about your son-in-law. My introductory sociology class is reading Heller's *Something Happened* this semester and one of the themes is that the system is run by fear. I couldn't help thinking that if I had read Dante during Dante's time, I'd have believed it. I would really be afraid too, to find what ring I was going to end up on. With respect to something you said earlier, Dr. Cain, you may recall some early works on social disorganization. In trying to explain delinquency it was argued that rites of passage were nonexistent in the legitimate structure of American society and so delinquent behavior became an alternative set of rites. So it is conceivable that if we follow this pattern of allowing a sufficient amount of space, that we might get a spontaneous organization of behavior on the part of the elderly. The only thing that concerns me is that the evidence shows that our society does not allow people to float around unintegrated. Dr. Monge talked about the intentionality of the people who make decisions about the Peace Corps. Piven and Cloward were able to really demonstrate the very strong plausibility of manipulation. In my study of the Federal Writers and Artists projects, I have Harry Hopkins and Roosevelt knowing precisely that they established the Writers and Artists project in order to get these people off the street corners. Similarly, the American Legion came into existence in 1919 because "the boys had been exposed to bolshevism in Europe." Teddy Roosevelt was behind that, and soon after they reached public awareness, they got rid of Roosevelt. They didn't want anybody to know that he had been involved with it. One of the interesting things about going off to war and going off on Crusades is you always took along your radicals. You never left them back on the farm because they'd take over. This suggests intentionality.

LOPATA: Would you clarify something for me on this question of abeyance? It seems to me that the function of abeyance structures may be either manifest or latent. I'm thinking here, in terms of a latent abeyance structure, the idea of secondary career orientations for women. Some occupations, especially female roles, facilitate that marginal status in between when you are too old to stay at home and not work and still have not found someone to marry yet.

MIZRUCHI: Yes. That's another one of these transitional kinds of things.

LOPATA: Just an interesting twist on this. Dr. Sheppard's questions about whether we should kick people out of the occupational work force to let young people in. The argument against that is that roughly a third of positions which become vacant through retirement are eliminated. In a sense, these positions are abeyance structures keeping people out of retirement. In other words, the job, the position is only being maintained in order to delay retirement.

MIZRUCHI: That's very interesting. There are other dynamics here. There are cases where people are pushed out, like Jews during the medieval period were pushed out of jobs to make jobs for non-Jews. In Everett Hughes,' "Good People and Dirty Work" about Nazi Germany this is one of the things that Hughes was really finding--people were telling him Jews were getting all the good jobs and things like that--somebody had to get rid of them.

Chapter 6 SCHEDULES AND SOCIAL CONTROL

Eviatar Zerubavel, Ph.D.
Department of Sociology
Columbia University

Time is one of the major parameters of the social world, and much of social life is structured and regulated in accordance with it. Man's growing independence of nature has by no means entailed independence of all temporal determinants of his activities, and even modern Western man, who has abandoned the traditional seasonally-based rural lifestyle, and has invented such technological facilities as the electric light and central heating to defy the night and the winter, has not yet fully liberated himself from all *temporal constraints*. In fact, I shall attempt to demonstrate here that, with respect to the temporal patterning of his life, man has only replaced natural control with social control.

The present paper brings into focus one of the cornerstones of the social order, namely the *"sociotemporal order."* It is the functional analogue of the "physiotemporal" and "biotemporal" orders which regulate the motion of celestial bodies and the lives of living organisms, and though, unlike them, it rests on social conventions rather than natural forces, it is by no means less constraining. As a "social fact,"[1] it is not only external to the individual, but also endowed with coercive power, which is felt mostly when one attempts to resist it, and by virtue of which it imposes itself on him and constrains him independently of his will.

However, we very rarely try to resist this order. Instead, we

*I feel particularly indebted to my friend and colleague Charles Lidz, who, with much patience, gave careful critical readings to several early versions of this paper.

usually take it for granted and use it as a basis for ordering our personal and social activities.

More specifically, the paper brings into focus the foremost institutionalized manifestation of the sociotemporal order in the modern Western world, namely the *schedule*. (I shall use this term in a generic sense, that is, as an "umbrella concept" which covers the institutions of the timetable and the calendar as well.) Being concerned here mainly with the regulative aspects of the sociotemporal order, and regarding the schedule as the main social institution in accordance with which modern social life is temporally structured, I shall discuss its function as a major agency of social control.

TEMPORAL REGULARITY

Much of the temporal organization of modern social life is based on forcing activities in a systematic way into rather rigid temporal patterns. This is actually accomplished by establishing *temporal regularity,* which is the fundamental principle underlying the schedule, and which at least one observer of modernity considered to be "The first characteristic of modern machine civilization."[2] Regarding *sequence, duration, timing,* and *tempo* as the fundamental parameters of schedules,[3] I view temporal regularity as a four-dimensional phenomenon, namely a routine association of activities or events with (a) rigid sequential orders, (b) fixed durations, (c) standard locations in time, and (d) uniform rates of recurrence.

In other words, I shall bring into focus four different aspects of the temporal regularity which underlies the modern sociotemporal order, namely the rigidification of the sequential order of social activities and events, the routinization of their durations, the standardization of their locations in time, and the uniformization of their rates of recurrence.

(a) *Rigid sequential orders.* The most elementary temporal structure conceivable is the sequential ordering of two events. It is in the nature of many social events and activities that they cannot all take place simultaneously and must, therefore, be temporally segregated from one another in terms of "before" and "after." While the temporal structure of such series of events or activities is sometimes purely random, there are many occasions whereby the sequential order in accordance with which they are arranged is rigid to the point of irreversibility. An integral part of the social world of everyday life,[4] rigid sequential structures are applied to simple procedural agendas (e.g. a conference's schedule) as well as imposed on entire lifetimes (e.g. marriage before procreation), not to mention, of course, routine daily, weekly, monthly, or annual schedules of all kinds. Though the routinized temporal relations among the various "structural slots" within military ceremonies, church services, "career timetables,"[5] or academic programs may suggest that they are particularly typical of formal organizational life, dating "norms of sequence"[6] imply that they govern even the more informal domains of social life.

(b) *Fixed durations.* Also characteristic of the modern Western sociotemporal order is the way in which social events are associated with certain fixed durations on a regular, routine basis. Consider, for example, the rigid definition of lectures as 60-minute events or vacations as three-week stretches of time. Much of the predictability in modern everyday life depends on "durational expectancies,"[7] which presuppose the durational rigidity of so many social activities. To take an example from a teaching hospital whose temporal organization I have studied,[8] "attending rounds" could be scheduled regularly for 10:00 a.m. only with the assurance that the morning round, which used to begin at 8:00 a.m., would not last for more than two hours.

Moreover, though it has never been stated anywhere that entertainment events ought to last for about two hours, there seems to be some tacit consensus, based on viewing the relation between social events and their routine durations as intrinsic, which would probably lead many people to feel cheated if a movie or concert for which they paid a full-price ticket would last for only ten minutes. The "only" here suggests that we have some pretty well defined notions of "proper durations," which, even though never formulated explicitly, are nevertheless normatively binding.

Consider, for example, the highly symbolic significance of leaving "too soon." On the other hand, that even very close friends are sometimes said to have stayed "too long" suggests that normative notions, as well as actual patterns, of durational rigidity exist even in the relatively unstructured realm of intimacy.

The major peculiarity of the durational rigidity which is characteristic of the modern Western sociotemporal order is that it is tied to a conception of time as a quantitative entity which is segmentable into various "quantities" of duration. In other words, the modern Western time units are "objectified as counted *quantities,* especially as lengths, made up of units as a length can be visibly marked off into inches."[9] Being perceived as "quantities," they are also characterized by being standard, that is, durationally uniform. Thus, whereas the length of the ancient Egyptian hour, for example, varied across seasons (being defined as one-twelfth of daylight time), the modern Western hour is always of the same standard "length," regardless of whether its measurement begins at 6:26 a.m. during the winter of 1993 in Norway or at 11:17 p.m. during the summer of 1654 in Sudan.

Similarly, as a "quantity" of duration, a year is socially regarded as a "year," whether it begins on January 1 (the Gregorian New Year's Day), July 1 (the beginning of a new annual cycle in teaching hospitals), the first week of September (the beginning of the academic year), or November 25 (my birthday).

That our time units are regarded as standard "quantities" of duration has been made possible by measuring them against the clock, which is paced at a uniform rate. The introduction of durational rigidity into modern Western social life would have been impossible without the notion of *clock time* (which may account, in part, for why Lewis Mumford regarded the clock as "the key machine of the modern industrial age"[10]).

It is this notion that made it possible for Western man "to fix time as something that happens between two points,"[11] as the durations measured by parking meters and stopwatches[12] seem to suggest. One of the major characteristics of modern

Western time units is that they are viewed as entirely abstract entities, utterly removed from, and not anchored in, any concrete context of events. As the measurement of time in chess, basketball, or football suggests, measured time may very well be even dissociated entirely from passing time. "Time assumes for us an autonomous character and we are free to manipulate temporal concepts instrumentally, without constant reference to specific events."[13]

Whereas a time unit as the solar tropical year is defined as a period contextually anchored in nature (namely as the time between two successive passages of the sun through the spring equinox), such clock-time units as the hour or the minute are purely abstract, since they exist only within clock time. Like language, clock time is a symbolic system whose elementary units--like words--have no intrinsic value of their own. Whatever meaning they have derives only from the system of which they are a part, since if it were not for that system, they would not even exist.

(c) *Standard locations in time.* In a way that suggests Ecclesiastes' doctrine that "To every thing there is a season, and a time to every purpose under the heaven," many social events and activities are also associated routinely with particular times of the day, days of the week, parts of the year, or periods in a person's lifetime, to a point where these periods are socially perceived as their natural and inevitable "containers." Thus, most offices open around 8:00 or 9:00 a.m. most people do not work on Sunday, schools usually begin around September, and women are expected to get married in their early twenties. On the other hand, it is almost inconceivable that a concert or a dancing party would be given in the morning or a Bar Mitzvah scheduled for Monday, and drinking alcohol at the age of 11 would be regarded as inappropriate, as well as illegal.

To fully appreciate the significance of the distinction between rigid scheduling and a spontaneous location of social events in time, note that, whereas modern Western parties are usually scheduled for a certain *fixed time of the day, many comparable events in other civilizations are geared to no schedule, and begin not at any pre-set time, but, rather, "when 'things' are ready.*"[14] This aspect of rigid scheduling is probably one of the key characteristics of social life in the modern West.

(d) *Uniform rates of recurrence.* The last aspect of temporal regularity is related to what various authors have referred to as the "rhythmic structure of social life."[15] The modern Western sociotemporal order presupposes various regularly recurrent patterns of social life. Such periodic patterns are regular not only in a social sense, as when family reunions are temporally spaced according to the rigid routine of "every wedding" or "every funeral," but also in a mathematical sense. Thus, there are many periodic social events which are temporally spaced at mathematically regular intervals.

Consider, for example, the annual celebration of holidays and birthdays, meetings that are held on a monthly basis, the weekly pattern of church attendance, or daily family dinners. It should be noted that the rigid rhythmicity which is imposed on social life by the temporal spacing of recurrent social events and activities at mathematically regular intervals is not characteristic only of formal organization. In the modern West, relatively uniform rates of recurrence of periodic social activities can be identified even within the relatively unstructured domain of informal relations. As the normative overtones of such notions as "too often" or "hardly ever" suggest, even the temporal spacing of "casual" visits, telephone calls, and exchanged letters among friends--which I consider to be a most adequate indicator of the "moral density"[16]of social relations--is very often regulated by some regular "proper tempi."

THE CONVENTIONALITY OF SCHEDULES

One fundamental characteristic of the sociotemporal order is that, unlike the "physiotemporal" and "biotemporal" orders, it is not a natural phenomenon, but, rather, a social artifact. In order to highlight this, I shall elaborate here on a theme that was originally introduced by Hubert and Mauss,[17] and later explored further by Sorokin,[18] namely the conventional and arbitrary basis of the temporal organization of social life.

One ought to realize, for example, that many rigid sequential structures which are usually seen as inevitable and unalterable nevertheless rest on social conventions alone. Of course, there are irreversibilities which are either determined by nature or logically or technically inevitable. It is a natural imperative, for example, that forces farmers to plow their fields before sowing; it is a logical necessity that forces track-meet organizers to schedule heats before finals; and it is a technical constraint that underlies the mixing of coffee only after cream and sugar have been added. There are also some sequentially rigid behavior patterns, like those habitualized by obsessive-compulsive persons as "personal rituals," which are purely psychological in origin. Yet such irreversibilities ought to be distinguished from those which are socially based. Not only is it just conventional to serve soup before, rather than after, meat; the very fact that the "Pennsylvania Dutch," for example, serve all their dishes simultaneously suggests the purely conventional basis of the entire institutionalization of temporally segregated "courses." Similarly, it is purely arbitrary social conventions that govern the temporal relations between nouns and adjectives (which accounts, for example, for the variation between the English and French languages). Likewise, while it is a technical constraint that imposes an irreversibility between the acts of putting on socks and shoes, it is basically a social convention that imposes one between the acts of putting on undershirts and shirts, as some circus clowns enjoy demonstrating. Finally, as I have shown elsewhere, though there are usually sound organizational rationales underlying the sequential rigidity of various routine bureaucratic procedures, it is by no means "natural" and inevitable, and the temporal structures of those procedures are very often actually altered and reversed.[19] Socially based irreversibilities are often purely symbolic in origin, as the sequential rigidity built into the schedules of weddings or commencement ceremonies seems to indicate.

The distinction between naturally- and socially-based sequential rigidity is probably most evident when one compares courtship rituals cross-specifically. Such a comparison may very well suggest where nature ends and society begins. Whereas the courtship ceremonies of water salamanders or sticklebacks generally consist of biologically determined "reaction chains," whereby each link in the chain functions as an almost indispensable "releaser" of the mate's next move (as, for example, a ritualized fanning by the male is needed in order to "release" the female's entrance to the nest),[20] human courtship rituals are culturally controlled. The "proper sequences" which underlie such normative prescriptions as "too early" often vary not only across cultures, but also across historical periods and age groups within each culture, and are of an almost purely symbolic significance.

Neither are many patterns of routinely associating particular social activities with particular fixed durations "natural" and inevitable, though they often appear to be so on the surface. Whereas the relative durational rigidity of a pregnancy period or an Amsterdam-Rome flight is pretty much biologically or technically determined, that of training programs, vacations, holidays, or examinations is purely conventional (though, as a "social fact," by no means less real). To appreciate the conventionality of the latter durations, note that they are actually alterable, as the practice of cutting down various training programs during wartime indicates. Note, also, that they are usually defined officially in terms of such "rounded quantities" of time as "three years" (or "six semesters"), "three weeks," "one day," or "two hours" (rather than, say, "nine days, six hours, thirty-seven minutes, and twenty-one seconds").

Similarly, in order to appreciate the conventionality of the routine location of particular social events in particular periods of time, note that scheduled events are usually set so as to begin at such "rounded" times as "on the hour," and that it is inconceivable that a dinner or a wedding would be scheduled for, say, "8:19 p.m." There has been a trend, in the West, of moving away from "the natural or casual sense of time towards a sense of time as schedule,"[21] whereby social activities are temporally located in accordance with a routine, fixed, pre-set conventional schedule, rather than either spontaneously or in accordance with nature. To realize the fundamental difference between naturally-determined and conventional patterns of locating events in time, contrast, for example, the reasons underlying sowing in spring or hunting during the daytime with those underlying going to church on Sunday or to college at the age of 18. That the standard temporal locations of so many social activities and events are only pseudo-natural becomes most evident when they are contrasted with timing patterns of pre-socialized infants, the retired aged, the unemployed, artists, shift workers, hippies, and members of other cultures.

The conventional basis of the routine tempi that govern social life is also suggested by their being associated with our standard units of time. Thus, for example, one would rather write to one's parents regularly every two weeks than, say, every sixteen days. Similarly, despite the strong biological basis of the temporal structure of the administration of medications in hospitals, their being regularly spaced at six- or four-hour intervals — rather than, say, at 4-hour-38-minute intervals — is basically supported by a social convention. Note, in this respect, that the standard cycles of the month, the year, and the day — not to mention, of course, the week and the hour, whose conventional basis is rather obvious — with which so many social periodicities are associated, are, at least in part, conventionally based. These cycles never correspond precisely to the periods of the moon's revolution around the earth and the latter's revolution around the sun and rotation on its own axis, respectively, but are, rather, "rounded" approximations of those. Moreover, even if these cycles did originally derive from natural periodicities, their very selection as the cornerstones of our sociotemporal order was in itself a matter of convention. It is only social convention that ties the spacing of holidays, pay days, geography classes, or coffee breaks to the year, the month, the week, and the day. Likewise, whereas the annual work/rest cycle of hunters is inherently associated with such natural periodic phenomena as seasonal variations in the availability of game, the association of young physicians' professional mobility with an annual rhythm is purely artificial.

In order to fully appreciate the artificial basis of the rigid rhythmicity imposed on social life, I should add that, not only is social rhythmicity so often independent of natural rhythmicity, it sometimes even conflicts with it. As we substitute "mechanical periodicity" for "organic periodicity,"[22] and free ourselves from submission to natural cycles, we increasingly risk internal disruption.[23] That we are so often sleepy when we have to get up and yet wide awake at bedtime, for example, may very well be a direct consequence of imposing a 24-hour rhythmicity, which derives from the adherence of our standard daily schedules to the conventional clock time, on our bodies, which are believed to be internally regulated by *circadian* rhythms (which, by definition, very rarely correspond precisely to our 24-hour days).

CONSTRAINT AND SOCIAL ORDER

That the temporal regularity built into our sociotemporal order often involves social constraint is already suggested by the sequential rigidification of social life. Worshippers, for example, have no choice whatever with regard to which stanza ought to be sung first in a hymn, and students must accept the bureaucratic rulings of academia which often make participation in one course a prerequisite for participation in another. The coercive element involved in the imposition of rigid sequential structures probably becomes even more evident when one considers the way some cultural moral codes forbid couples to experience sexual intimacy before going through an official wedding ceremony.

The coercive aspect of temporal regularity is also very evident with respect to the durational rigidification of social life. As soldiers in basic training learn how to finish their breakfast within a fixed number of minutes, so do hospital patients learn to adhere to the durational rigidity of visiting hours, and students that they must respect that of examinations. Consider, also, the case of speaking time in conferences, whereby speakers who are supposed to deliver a "one-hour presentation" are expected to talk for about an hour, regardless of whether they may have much more or much less to present. Durational flexibility, on the other hand, is symbolically associated with freedom. It was typical of the late sixties, for example, that rock concerts used to last much longer than conventional concerts, and that their organizers refused to adhere to an externally imposed durational rigidification of artistic events and experiences.

Controlling the temporal location of one's activities against one's will also involves much constraint. While this is very obvious in the case of imposed curfews,[24] it is by no means less true in the case of the introduction of daylight saving time by various governments. While coercion may be manifested in a total randomization of the temporal location of one's activities (as when prisoners are ordered to perform certain chores in accordance with no schedule at all), it is nevertheless usually exercised by standardizing it, that is, by routinely associating those activities with particular fixed times of the day, days of the week, periods in one's lifetime, and so on. Hence the resistance of most modern bureaucracies to flexible work schedules, as well as their constant struggle to preserve standard retirement age. Consider also, in this respect, the very striking phenomenon of the socially-based synchronizaton of collective sentiments by the calendar, as in the institutionalization of holidays and memorial days,[25] for example. An extreme case, such as the calendrical fixing of the Israeli National Memorial Day and Independence Day immediately next to one another, seems to suggest that the collective "mood" of an entire society[26] can actually be steered so as to switch, at the sound of a siren, from one extreme emotional state to its diametrical opposite.

But most striking, probably, is the way in which biological activities are structured in accordance with a sociotemporal, rather than any "biotemporal," order. Thus, for example, it is conventional sociocultural normative notions of "proper timing," rather than any biological imperatives, that compel one to rest on weekends or avoid any sexual intercourse during particular phases of one's menstrual cycle. The coercive aspect of this was noted already two thousand years ago:

The gods confounded the man who first found out
How to distinguish hours — confounded him, too,
Who in this place set up a sun-dial,
To cut and hack my days so wretchedly

Into small pieces! When I was a boy,
My belly was my sun-dial—one more sure,
Truer, and more exact than any of them.
This dial told me when 'twas proper time
To go to dinner, when I ought to eat;
But, now-a-days, why even when I have,
I can't fall to unless the sun gives leave.
The town's so full of these confounded dials.[27]

In fact, imposing the conventional daily schedule on one's internal "biological clock" is one of the very first stages of primary socialization, and the daily conflicts between parents and children over mealtimes and bedtime are most indicative of its coercive aspect. Actually, bedtime is symbolically associated with privileged social rank, and children's gradual promotion to a later bedtime, and eventually to attainment of total control over it, is a part of a symbolic process of their maturation.[28]

Finally, to appreciate the coercive aspect of the uniformization of the rates of recurrence of social events, note that the cycles with which they are associated not only mark periodical social patterns, but, very often, actually create them! As Durkheim so brilliantly commented, the calendar not only expresses the rhythm of social life, but also functions as assurer of the regular recurrence of periodical social events as rites, feasts, and such public ceremonies as prayers or holidays.[29] It is very significant to note, in this respect, that in two of the most notable attempts in modern Western history to challenge the Church's control of social life, namely the French and the Soviet revolutions, there were considerable efforts to control the rhythm of collective life by abolishing the religiously grounded seven-day week and replacing it by a different social cycle.[30] Both revolutions aimed deliberately at disrupting the traditional church-attending practices by introducing new collective rhythms which presented enormous practical, as well as cognitive, difficulties in keeping up with the traditional seven-day cycle. Had these attempts succeeded, it would have been most difficult to live in accordance with a seven-day cycle within a society which adhered to a ten-day or a five-day week. (That a Robinson

Crusoe would still keep track of the days of the week far away from civilization is highly suggestive of the coercive power of standard collective rhythms once internalized.)

It is hardly surprising, therefore, that the schedule, the calendar, the timetable, and the clock have been regarded by many as actual oppressors which regiment individuals' lives. Lewis Mumford's classic critique of the temporal regularity associated with the introduction of clock time[31] is a famous case in point. The schedule has also been portrayed as an agent representing compelling external forces, and the adherence to it associated with repressive toilet training.[32] Lawrence Wright went as far as identifying man's subservience to timekeeping ("chronarchy") as one of the themes most characteristic of the modern Western world.[33] The association of temporal regularity with the order of repression is even more pronounced in various radical writings. Woodcock, for example, regarded the clock as an inhibitor of man's actions, and condemned "this slavish dependence on mechanical time" as responsible for bringing about "the demoralizing regimentation of life," adding that "Socially the clock had a more radical influence than any other machine, in that it was the means by which the regularization and regimentation of life necessary for an exploiting system of industry could best be attained."[34] Such arguments gain much support from the fact that many people, especially when on vacation, display a symbolic defiance of external control by deliberately not wearing a watch.

However, social control implies much more than mere repression. In fact, I would like to argue that modern Western social life in general would have been impossible without the institutionalization of some element of temporal regularity. Coordinating the timing of various people's activities becomes necessary if a group of them is to be brought together for a planned meeting, and the indispensability of the schedule becomes even more evident when we consider the high degree of differentiation within modern social networks. As Simmel noted already at the turn of the century:

> The relationships and affairs of the typical

metropolitan are so varied and complex that without
the strictest punctuality in promises and services the
whole structure would break down into an inextricable
chaos. Above all, this necessity is brought about by the
aggregation of so many people with such differentiated
interests, who must integrate their relations and activities into a highly complex organism. . . Thus, the
technique of metropolitan life is unimaginable without
the most punctual integration of all activities and
mutual relations into a stable and impersonal time
schedule.[35]

As far as the sequential rigidification of social life is concerned, consider also how functionally essential *queuing* is to
social organization.[36] The institutionalization of turntaking is
necessary for the regulation of access to social goods. If two
persons engage in a conversation, they cannot both talk simultaneously, and each of them must give up the floor from time to
time. Similarly, if they play chess, their respective moves must
be made one at a time. The institution of the *deadline* is functionally similar, as far as the durational rigidification of social
life is concerned. Modern social life as we know it would have
been impossible, for example, were surgeons, newspaper re-
porters, secretaries, or police investigators to carry on their
assigned tasks indefinitely.

The rather rigid temporal patterning of social life provides
not only for a highly structured organizational order, but for a
highly reliable cognitive order as well. In other words, aside
from their regulative function as sort of traffic lights which
coordinate various social actors' activities, schedules also
answer the basic psychological need for some structure, thus
safeguarding against cognitive anomie. As far as predictability
is concerned, for example, the rather rigid temporal regularities
on which our sociotemporal order is based provide a sort of
"repertoire" of what is expected, possible, or unlikely within
certain temporal boundaries (which accounts for the fact that
schedules are usually placed in central locations). It is typical
that upon being asked where her boss was, a secretary once

replied: "I'll go and see what his calendar says." Temporal regularities also provide individuals with some normative prescriptions and standards which save them such questions as how long they ought to stay, what they should do next, or when they should pray. In general, many people feel uncomfortable without any rigid temporal constraints, and if these are not imposed on them by some external factor, they very often tend to impose them on themselves in order to be able to function efficiently.

Certainly not all modern social life is temporally patterned to such a rigid extent, yet temporal regularity is undoubtedly among the major characteristics of the modern Western world. The schedules which are based on it underlie some highly structured order which governs our life. Like many other "social facts," it is primarily the invisibility of the sociotemporal order that makes it so fascinating for the sociologist to unravel. It is one of those invisible phenomena that are usually taken for granted and, therefore, ignored, and yet which give such an unmistakable characteristic structure to modern social life.

FOOTNOTES

[1]Durkheim, 1964b:1-13.
[2]Mumford, 1934:269.
[3]Zerubavel, 1976:88-90. See also Lauer, 1973:452.
[4]Berger and Luckmann, 1967:27-28.
[5]Roth, 1963.
[6]Lyman and Scott, 1970:195-97.
[7]Toffler, 1971:42-44.
[8]Zerubavel, forthcoming.
[9]Whorf, 1956:140.
[10]Mumford, 1934:14.
[11]McLuhan, 1964:135.
[12]Note, for example, that the notion of clock time is responsible for the introduction of timed records to sports, along with the very modern distinction between a "champion," which involves beating others, and a "record holder," which implies only beating the clock.
[13]Hallowell, 1937:669. Note, for example, how, by viewing time in terms of "quantities" of duration which are subject to mathematical operations, we allow for the addability, divisibility, or interchangeability of time periods. Thus, we

often add up "chunks" of time which are not temporally juxtaposed in actual reality, as when saying that someone has had "75 hours" of psychoanalysis, or when taping a 60-minute cassette which actually consists of two separate tapings (13:16 and 46:44 minutes long, respectively). Similarly, people sometimes "split up" a 21-day annual vacation into three seven-day segments which are taken off separately. One-hour appointments or lectures are also "moved" from one day to another and eight-hour shifts "switched" over between co-workers, as if those time periods were really "the same." In one extreme case, I have seen a nurse "moving" her "holiday time" so that she officially celebrated the Fourth of July on the twenty-ninth of July!

[14]Hall, 1959:22. See also Hallowell, 1937:657.

[15]Durkheim, 1965:23, 32n, 391, 488; Sorokin, 1941:542-51; Hawley, 1950:288-316; Kolaja, 1969.

[16]Durkheim, 1964a:257ff.

[17]Hubert and Mauss, 1909:213-19.

[18]Sorokin and Merton, 1937; Sorokin, 1941:542-51; Sorokin, 1943.

[19]Zerubavel, 1977b.

[20]Eibl-Eibesfeldt, 1970:184-90.

[21]Wax, 1960:452.

[22]Mumford, 1934:197:98.

[24]Lynch, 1972:75.

[25]Warner, 1962.

[26]Durkheim, 1965:442-49

[27]Plautus, cited in Wright, 1968:29.

[28]Aubert and White, 1959; Schwartz, 1970

[29]Durkheim, 1965:23.

[30]Zerubavel, 1977a; Moore, 1963:122.

[31]Mumford, 1934:12-18, 269-71.

[32]Wright, 1968:213; Meerloo, 1966:249.

[33]Wright, 1968:213-19.

[34]Woodcock, 1944:265-66.

[35]Simmel, 1950:412-13.

[36]Schwartz, 1975.

BIBLIOGRAPHY

Aubert, V., and H. White. 1959. "Sleep: A Sociological Interpretation." *Acta Sociologica* 4:1-16.

Berger, Peter L., and Thomas Luckmann. 1967. *The Social Construction of Reality*. Garden City: Anchor Books.

Durkheim, Emile. 1964a. *The Division of Labor in Society*. New York: The Free Press.

Durkheim, Emile. 1964b. *The Rules of Sociological Method*. New York: The Free Press.

Durkheim, Emile. 1965. *The Elementary Forms of the Religious Life*. New York: The Free Press.

Eibl-Eibesfeldt, Irenäus. 1970. *Ethology*. New York: Holt, Rinehart and Winston, Inc.

Hall, Edward T. 1959. *The Silent Language*. New York: Premier Books.

Hallowell, Irving. 1937. "Temporal Orientation in Western Civilization and in a Pre-Literate Society." *American Anthropologist* 39:647-70.

Hawley, Amos H. 1950. *Human Ecology*. New York: The Ronald Press Co.

Hubert, Henri, and Marcel Mauss. 1909. "Étude Sommaire de la Représentation du Temps dans la Magie et la Religion." Pp. 189-229 in *Mélanges d'Histoire des Religions*. Paris: Librairies Félix Alcan et Guillaumin Réunies.

Kolaja, Jiri. 1969. *Social System and Time and Space*. Pittsburgh: Duquesne University Press.

Lauer, Robert H. 1973. "Temporality and Social Change." *Sociological Quarterly* 14:451-64.

Lyman, Stanford M., and Marvin B. Scott. 1970. "On the Timetrack." Pp. 189-212 in *A Sociology of the Absurd*. New York: Appleton-Century-Crofts.

Lynch, Kevin. 1972. *What Time is This Place?* Cambridge: MIT Press.

McLuhan, Marshall. 1964. *Understanding Media*. New York: Signet Books.

Meerloo, Joost A. M. 1966. "The Time Sense in Psychiatry." Pp. 235-52 in *The Voices of Time*. Ed. Julius Thomas Fraser. New York: George Braziller.

Moore, Wilbert E. 1963. *Man, Time, and Society*. New York: John Wiley.

Mumford, Lewis. 1934. *Technics and Civilization*. New York: Harcourt, Brace, and World.

Roth, Julius A. 1963. *Timetables*. Indianapolis: The Bobbs-Merrill Co., Inc.

Schwartz, Barry. 1970. "Notes on the Sociology of Sleep." *Sociological Quarterly* 11:485-99.

Schwartz, Barry. 1975. *Queuing and Waiting*. Chicago and London: The University of Chicago Press.

Simmel, Georg. 1950. *The Sociology of Georg Simmel*. Ed. Kurt H. Wolff. New York: The Free Press.

Sorokin, Pitirim A. 1941. *Social and Cultural Dynamics, Vol. IV*. New York: The Bedminster Press.

Sorokin, Pitirim A. 1943. *Sociocultural Causality, Space, Time*. Durham: Duke University Press.

Sorokin, Pitirim A., and Robert K. Merton. 1937. "Social Time: A Methodological and Functional Analysis." *American Journal of Sociology* 42:615-29.

Toffler, Alvin. 1971. *Future Shock*. New York: Bantam.

Warner, W. Lloyd. 1962. "An American Sacred Ceremony." Pp. 5-34 in

American Life: Dream and Reality. Chicago: The University of Chicago Press.

Wax, Murray. 1960. "Ancient Judaism and the Protestant Ethic." *American Journal of Sociology* 65:449-55.

Whorf, Benjamin Lee. 1956. "The Relation of Habitual Thought and Behavior to Language." Pp. 134-59 in *Language, Thought and Reality*. Ed. John B. Carroll. Cambridge: MIT Press.

Woodcock, George. 1944. "The Tyranny of the Clock." *Politics* 1:265-67.

Wright, Lawrence. 1968. *Clockwork Man*. London: Elek Books.

Zerubavel, Eviatar. 1976. "Timetables and Scheduling: On the Social Organization of Time." *Sociological Inquiry* 46:87-94.

Zerubavel, Eviatar. 1977a. "The French Republican Calendar: A Case Study in the Sociology of Time." *American Sociological Review* 42:868-77.

Zerubavel, Eviatar. 1977b. "The Temporal Structure of Psychiatric Procedures: Informed Consent and the Temporal Location of Decisions." Paper presented at the Annual Meetings of the American Psychiatric Association, Toronto.

Zerubavel, Eviatar. Forthcoming. *Patterns of Time*.

K. MARSHALL: You said the watch, the wrist watch, was an agent of social control that we carry on our body. For a person in a temporally regimented, synchronized society, the wrist watch also represents a kind of unique opportunity for individual freedom, as well as the individual's opportunity to synchronize himself with the society so as to maximize his own goals regardless of the potential cost to society.

ZERUBAVEL: He doesn't have a choice. You won't adjust your watch so that it will show a time three hours different from that of other watches and clocks in your time zone.

K. MARSHALL: No, one does not adjust one's watch but by knowing what time it is at any given time, by knowing what time it is to the rest of that society and then can exploit that knowledge. One can avoid circumstances, such as the burglar who is seeking to avoid when the policeman makes his rounds.

ZERUBAVEL: The burglar is still controlled by the temporal patterns of the policeman. He has to adjust to the policeman rather than the other way around.

SCHWARTZ: Social organization is itself a clock because it's a reliable, regularly recurring process. It's a social clock, a process out there, in the same sense that a clock is an object out there. And it's a process to which people gear their activities. It isn't a process that determines the activities; it's a process that people take into account as they formulate their separate courses of action. The schedule is something that can be employed in pursuit of their own interests. For example, schedules are often used to dramatize power, as with a supervisor who comes into work before he has to, to dramatize his greater commitment to the job than his subordinates. As far as duration is concerned, often the length of a training period will be constructed with the view to maintaining a monopoly on a practice of some kind. Dentistry is an excellent example. During World War II we trained the kids to pull teeth within a very short period of time--six weeks, eight weeks. Our dental schools require we go four years now. So here's an instance in which people put these tools you would call "hard," "rigid," "regimenting" and so forth to their own use.

What seems to me to best point out the inherent flexibility of the scheduling control systems is that sanctions have to be employed in order to ensure that people are punctual. If people were intrinsically disposed to be punctual, then the sanctions themselves would be superfluous. But in fact we go to great pains to ensure that our children are punctual. On report cards, for example, there's one corner for days absent and the times tardy. It seems to me that you kind of painted yourself into a corner by perhaps over emphasizing the rigidity and the uncompromising qualities, the totalitarian character of control systems. Even the most totalitarian control systems, when you look at them closely, usually include very generous spans of various kinds.

ZERUBAVEL: I agree, and still if I had to present this again I would still present it this way for purely heuristic reasons, to show a certain direction that the program can take, though I could write a complementary paper. The fact, though, that it is flexible goes with what I said before: that since it's conventional the irreversibilities are only apparently irreversible. They are alterable, though they appear not to be.

V. MARSHALL: It is fallacious to say that a watch is an agent of social control. That's a reification of the first order. We often use watches ourselves--watches don't use us. We've all had the experience when someone's in our office, of wanting to get rid of them. We start glancing at our watch and finally they take the hint. I think the dimensions that you've outlined are very useful and could usefully be applied for example, to Glazer and Strauss' notion of status passage or to notions of careers. But the reason I thought of Glazer and Strauss is that they make the same error in their book on status passages, one of the properties of which, of course, is the temporal set of properties. They have this notion of a combative situation where some party or agent is always trying to control the inductee, whereas in fact a lot of people mutually or collaboratively fit lines of action together and coordinate their activities. My question is, or my thought that I pass on to you, is it really always control or is it often times coordination? Do we not often use these different dimensions in very creative ways?

ZERUBAVEL: Let me say two things. First, that I wanted to emphasize this dimension and neglect entirely the second one for heuristic purposes of demonstrating it. If I were giving a general presentation on calendars or schedules and social control I emphasize this, of course. But the other thing is that whenever you think of social control systems there's always this leeway. Look, a child is put to bed by his parents, they close the door and there is darkness and then the child does whatever he wants to do in the darkness. Now does it mean that he's not socially controlled? You say that we use the clock. Sure we use the clock. We sometimes use our supervisors for our own purposes. Now does it mean that we're not controlled by them? I don't think it's a problem with this analysis but a problem with what social control is.

SCHWARTZ: My wife and I have established in over seven years of marriage a lot of routines, temporal routines, but they're agreements. We have expectations that I'm going to get up first and things like that. I'm not controlling her and she's not controlling me. We're coordinating lines of activity. Lots of the uses of time are not coercive.

ZERUBAVEL: O.K., but I started with Durkheim's notion of social facts. I'm talking about coercion with his notion that social facts are constraining. As Durkheim pointed out, you don't notice the coercion until people try to resist it. When you try and you can't or you can with difficulties or with sanctions, then you feel that it is coercive. I am not suggesting that you look at the world from a strategic Machiavellian point of view. I am suggesting that there is this social control we may be totally unaware of, and that we notice it when we try to resist it. If you try one of these mornings, if you have these routines, if you really felt that you wanted to stay in bed but you can't because you have to get out of bed, then you feel that you are controlled. I think that you are socially controlled. The fact that you are a part of it does not mean that the social part of you did not control the other part in you.

CAIN: I'll try to be very brief. I do not have a criticism but an application I think for gerontology. Recently a student of mine submitted a little narrative that went like this, on why Mrs. M did not make the doctor's appointment yesterday. This man is a bus driver--he runs mini-buses. He goes around and picks up five or six older people to get them to their doctors' appointments. Mrs. M was first on the list and she was there promptly on her front porch at 2:00 p.m. and got on the bus. The doctor's appointment is an hour and a half later. But three or four or five people picked up in the interim produced the problem. There is another little lady who fears incontinency and she waits until the bus comes up, then goes back to the bathroom for five minutes. Then there is the person who is idiosyncratic--you don't know whether he will be anxious to get on beforehand and will come early and stand in the rain or will be in the house and have to be persuaded to leave. The bus driver is faced with this decision-- on the one hand there is the moral imperative to give full deference to every older person. You let that older person express his or her individuality--to be afraid of incontinence, to be this or that. But when you do that Mrs. M., the first one who is on the list, invariably gets shortchanged. And so the question becomes how to apply the notion of duration and have social control over the people, and which people, and how so.

HALL: I have no particular appreciation of Durkheim because I think he leaves a lot out, and yet I appreciate your sticking to your guns with him because I think you're right: we have to face up to social control and its relationship to time, independently of all the qualifications that people could make about cases where it doesn't occur. You really tap into the cases in which it does. But the Durkheimian problem is that it treats these social facts as God-given or systematically-given or whatever. You have to look at two questions beyond Durkheim: First, who is benefiting from and who is implementing the social control, and implementing domination--they are two different things and you are confusing them. It is true that time, like language, is an intersubjective element par excellence. If I want to speak to you so that you understand me, I will not speak Swahili to you, unless you understand Swahili. In this sense I am then oppressed by my language if I wish to speak to anybody but myself. In some sense you could even say, and I mean this not in a phenomenological-philosophical sense but in a psychological sense, I'm oppressed by language even when I speak to myself, because I have to create categories. But then this is the Durkheimian sense of coercion. There is another form of coercion, as when I stick a gun up to our legal expert here and say, "Give me your money," or when we seek domination socially. That form of coercion I believe is historically where you are mistaken. Schedules are one of the great democratizing principles of history. Schedules constitute the introduction of equality by permitting demands to be identified and regulated and rejected. Prior to the introduction of time if you were a laborer prior to the 17th century in Britain, you were owned by the man for whom you worked and fortunately Sunday was the one day on which no demands could be made upon you. In the 19th century there was the great reserve army of labor, where there was no five day work week. A man worked two days, three days, possibly he might work a week, then the market would decline; he would not work for six weeks, would not work for two weeks, then work for two days more. That man could not leave for fear of not being able to make money. With the introduction of schedules it became possible to say, "No, after 5:00 it is my time. You cannot ask me to do that." Schedules constitute attributing significance to an individual. A way of saying this is that when your time is not valuable, no one schedules it. Who is not scheduled in modern society? The poor.

ZERUBAVEL: I really have to disagree with you. I think an important point is that the very important people in our society make their own schedules, and if they are scheduled they are scheduled very precisely so that their time is used efficiently, because they are being paid a great deal of money. And the very poor are regimented into timetables and schedules, but those timetables and schedules are kept very loose and their own time, their own freedom is greatly restricted because of the very loose time schedule in which their office operates.

HALL: You misunderstand. I am not trying to say that everyone is equal because of a schedule. There is social differentiation. An impedement to the even greater exploitation of the social differentiation historically has been the implementation of schedules.

ZERUBAVEL: I see both sides of the coin. As I said, I mentioned here only one side just to answer the other side of the coin. I have written a paper trying to deal with time as a dimension of regulating social accessibility and I have made the distinction between private time and public time, taking the case of work schedules and showing the distinction between the doctor's work schedule and the nurse's work schedule and the nurse is precisely the one who has these rigid temporal boundaries over her public time, and the moment that she finishes giving her report she does not have to be there, that's the other side of the coin, yes.

SCHWARTZ: I got to thinking about Etzioni's compliance theory, and some of Everett Hughes' work, too, where they divide organizations according to the mechanisms of compliance, including utilitarian and renumerative types of control, normative controls, coercive controls, and so forth. I was wondering what the structural conditions of social organizations or societies would be which would determine how people respond differently to social control, or the structural conditions of society which would lead to different mechanisms for coordinating us around temporal schedules. I think it might be an interesting thing for someone as well versed in the area as yourself to consider. I do not think we have time now to deal with it. The question is how we are to characterize control systems in general. When we talk about bands of tolerance, when we talk about parents, when we talk about indulgence, we are talking about exceptions or "qualifications." We are talking about remissions which are an intrinsic part of the control system itself. Indeed the remissions are essential, they are instrumental to the controls or to the interdictions or to the constraints or whatever you want to call them. That is to say, the coercive function or aspect of the control system cannot operate effectively without the remissive characteristic, that is, without the band of tolerance. Now, if you want to cast this in a Durkheimian framework, you recall in Durkheim's discussion in *The Elementary Forms of the Religious Life,* how a very highly ritualized society suddenly goes to hell--all hell breaks loose. There is a periodic remission at which time all the conventional rules and standards go by the board.

ZERUBAVEL: It is nevertheless scheduled, right?

SCHWARTZ: Of course. But controls would be oppressive in the absence of these remissive elements. In their absence the control system itself would break down. It seems to me that what you have done is to emphasize the coercive. You focus on just one part of a control system which is essentially dialectic in nature. And by failing to sensitize yourself and us to the remissive aspects of control systems, we at the same time fail to appreciate how the controls can be maintained over time.

7 TIME'S RITE OF PASSAGE:
FROM INDIVIDUAL TO
SOCIETY

J. T. Fraser, D.Sc.
International Society for the
Study of Time.

This paper deals with the crisis in the balance between the
individual and collective identities of man as I see that crisis develop in our epoch. The arguments are based on the "theory of
time as a hierarchy of creative conflicts" that I have put forth
and elaborated elsewhere.[1]

1. THE TIME AND TIMES OF MATTER, ANIMALS, AND MAN

The theory of time as conflict sees the basic matrix of the
world as an open-ended hierarchy of integrative levels, each
with its peculiar temporality, causation, language, and unresolvable conflicts. The reasoning of this section is heavy on natural philosophy, extending to, but not seriously penetrating the
collective problems of sociotemporality.

It was over half a century ago that the German biologist
Jakob von Uexkull outlined his *Umweltlehre* or, in free translation, his principle of species-specific universes. He noted that an
animal's receptors determine its world of possible stimuli, its effectors the world of possible actions. Thus, for each animal the
world as perceived, together with the world as it might be acted
upon, is delimited by the possible functions of its effectors and
receptors. He called this world, carved out of the totality of the
animal's enivronment (as that is perceived by us) the animal's

Umwelt. What is not within an animal's *Umwelt* must be understood as not existing in its world.

For several reasons I retained the use of this German word but I enlarged its meaning substantially. The idea of umwelts may be easily formulated for specific sensory systems, then extended to the instruments of experimental science and eventually to the principles and equations of theoretical science. If, after thorough inquiry, a domain of nature is revealed to us consistently and exclusively only through a certain type of formalism, and if the appropriate abstract devices cannot accommodate certain features of the world which we ordinarily take for granted (or else, make familiar features appear in strange guise) then that domain of nature to which the formalism applies must be regarded as a distinct umwelt. I call this epistemic stance "the extended umwelt principle."[2]

There is a particular division of nature which I found very useful. It consists of the recognition of certain semi-autonomous integrative levels, that is, of certain groups of things and processes which display a great degree of unity, or wholeness, on some suitably selected scale.

In this scheme the basic substratum of the world is the integrative level of massless particles that travel at the speed of light. Above that level I perceive the world of elementary particles with non-zero mass, above this the astronomical universe of matter bunched into heavy masses that form stars, star clusters, galaxies, and clusters of galaxies. On a spherical object near one of the stars there evolved the integrative level of life, out of the many forms of life came human life characterized by a particular control that I shall call noetic. The highest integrative level known is that of civilizations and cultures, I shall call it the societal level. Each of these integrative levels may be identified as a distinct umwelt; each has its peculiar temporality. I shall now describe these temporalities in their simplest, paradigmatic forms.

The world of massless particles is *atemporal.* By this is meant that there are no ways whereby the hallmarks of time (future-past-present, before-after) may be recognized, if this world is judged entirely from within. The primitive time of the particulate umwelt I called *prototemporal* for "proto-" the first or lowest of a series. In a prototemporal umwelt distinction can be made between temporal and spatial features, even though our ideas of "here" vs. "there" and "now" vs. "then" are only loosely applicable. Causation is probabilistic, events can be described only statistically.

The Newtonian universe of massive, astronomical bodies is *eotemporal*, implying the dawn of time (for Eos, the Goddess of dawn). There is nothing in this world that could help us distinguish happenings that "flow" from past to future, from those that "flow" from future to past and, as in the atemporal and prototemporal worlds, nothing can correspond to our ideas of a "now." In this world causation is deterministic.

Living matter has its own umwelt, the *biotemporal*. It is only here that presentness becomes definable (in terms of the coordination necessary to maintain the autonomy of a living organism). We observe a series of "presents" as we progress from the primitive and cyclic to the complex and aging orders of life. Futurity and pastness become increasingly polarized and final causation can be given a meaning.

The umwelt of the mind I called *nootemporal*. This is the world of personal identity, and of signs and symbols. There is a sharp distinction between pastness and futurity; here the biotemporal present of animals opens up to the mental present of man with its continuously changing boundaries. Causality is enlarged to include human freedom.

The umwelt of a (potential) global collective of man may be called *sociotemporal*.

At this point reference should be made to Table I. It identifies the stable integrative levels of nature that I have mentioned, gives a description of their respective temporalities, and lists the paradigmatic and some other examples. To the content of that Table we may add that just as every integrative level subsumes those underneath it, so each temporality is taken to subsume the temporalities beneath it.

In the theory of time as conflict each major integrative level is further identified with certain *unresolvable conflicts*. By "unresolvable" is meant that through functions available within

Table 1. THE HIERARCHY OF TEMPORALITIES

Stable Integrative Levels of Nature	Temporalities and their Descriptions	Paradigms and Other Examples
First signals	ATEMPORAL. No before/after, no future/past/present.	Paradigm: the umwelt of particles with zero restmass. Other examples: physical, physiological and perceptual chronons.
Particulate matter.	PROTOTEMPORAL. Temporal and spatial positions of events ill-defined. Events and things sometimes interchangeable. Causation is probabilistic.	Paradigm: the umwelt of indistinguishable particles, such as all electrons. Other examples: all universes whose elements are countable but not orderable by numbers such as all workers in a factory, all voters above 18 years of age, all light bulbs. Also, the domain of time perception above the perceptual chronon but below the order threshold.
Ponderable matter.	EOTEMPORAL. Pure succession: not everything happens at once yet time does not have an arrow; endings cannot be distinguished from beginnings; connections are by deterministic causation.	Paradigm: the umwelt of the Newtonian world of heavy, gravitating bodies. Other examples: all universes whose elements are orderable by number but do not constitute autonomous systems that would command internal coordination such as: repetitive squences of a dance, periodic motion of the planets; the domain of the perception above the order threshold but below the threshold of conscious action dream imagery that contains future, past and

Table 1. THE HIERARCHY OF TEMPORALITIES *(Contd.)*

Stable Integrative Levels of Nature	Temporalities and their Descriptions	Paradigms and Other Examples
		present all at once yet unwinds "in time."
Life.	BIOTEMPORAL. Nowness may be defined; future may be distinguished from past, endings from beginnings. Connecticities may be those of final causation.	Paradigm: the umwelt of living organisms. Other examples: the mood of literary and artistic creations that suggest the emergence of presentness.
Mind.	NOOTEMPORAL. Future and past may be sharply distinguished; nowness is that of the mental present; connectivities include human freedom.	Paradigm: the umwelt of the human mind. Other examples: none known, but in principle all universes that comprise the symbolic transformations of experience.
Society.	SOCIOTEMPORAL. The possible features of this temporality, but mainly the reasons why it is difficult to delineate them, are argued in this paper.	Paradigm and only example: the (potential) global society of man.

that umwelt, the conflict may only be maintained or else eliminated by collapse into a lower integrative level. But, since the integrative level lasts only as long as the conflicts last, the collapse of the conflicts does not truly constitute their resolution. However, the unresolvable conflicts of a level can and do provide the motive forces for the emergence of a new integrative level. This new umwelt, from its very inception, may again be identified with certain unresolvable conflicts of its own.

There are, however, classes of phenomena which do not seem to belong in any of the major integrative levels but fall in between adjacent temporal umwelts. These phenomena determine conditions in nature which may be described as "interfaces." One sympathetic and knowledgeable critic found this feature of the theory important enough to remark that "nature does not make jumps, they used to say, but if you look at the hierarchy of complexity she seems not to linger at intermediate stages." I believe that the position of man in our epoch is at such an intermediate stage between the integrative level that corresponds to his individuality and one that corresponds to that of the family of man wherein individuals are significant only by virtue of their role in the communal enterprise. Let us, therefore, turn to a discussion of the interfaces, that is, to conditions and processes which, in the past, have given rise to new temporal umwelts. From what we shall have learned we will then extrapolate to time's rite of passage from the nootemporal to the sociotemporal.

2. POLICIES COMMON TO THE INTERFACES

It is not necessary to hypothesize the existence of interfaces between distinct integrative levels just to be able to discuss evolution. Throughout nature we may observe many examples of the emergence of the unpredictably new, well within the confines of the stable integrative levels. Thus, for instance, new elements have arisen from the primordial elements keeping totally within the physical integrative levels. Innumerable life forms have arisen totally within the integrative level of life. A rather impressive store of new ideas have arisen from the individual minds of people, properly classifiable as all within the nootemporal integrative level.

However, it is only from conditions and functions that we shall class as belonging to the interfaces that new temporal umwelts seem to arise. It is precisely this emergence of new temporalities that I describe by the phrase: time's rite of passage.

Let me now state without detailed arguments what I regard to be the distinguishing features of all interfaces taken as a group. But I shall do so only for the interfaces up through that between life and mind that is, the biotemporal and the nootemporal. Only later shall I attempt to apply what we have learned to the interface between individual and society.

Those structures and processes in nature which populate the interfaces may sometimes be classed as appropriate to a specific integrative level, sometimes to the level beneath it. Figuratively speaking, they are disowned by both of their adjacent, stable umwelts. By a term borrowed from chemistry I shall describe their positions along the evolutionary ladder as *metastable*. Upon close argument a case for metastability may be made for the "unpopularity" of atomic states which would separate the massless particles from those with finite masses and thus the atemporal from the prototemporal level; and again, for aggregate states that would be neither prototemporal nor eotemporal. Between the eotemporal and the biotemporal umwelts the region of biogenesis is certainly metastable; between the biotemporal and the nootemporal worlds we recognize a region of our functions which are too biological for the mind, as it were, and too tenuous and alien to the body: these are the unconscious manifestations of our minds.

Evolution has shown great ingenuity in finding *new uses for the functions and structures* of an integrative level, and through this policy it succeeded in determining the features of more advanced umwelts. Biogenesis is a rich example of this policy. All the elements that are necessary for primitive life must be assumed to have existed when life was born, but it is the new uses of already existing elements and compounds which is one of life's distinguishing features.[3] Equally rich in example is the interface between the biotemporal and the nootemporal. For instance, the nervous system, which is employed by animals mainly for the control of locomotion and communication, evolved into the human brain with functions of a much more complex nature. The auditory loop which, in animals, assists the survival of the species by means such as the blending of individual sensitivity to friend, foe, and food into collective sensitivities evolved, in man, into the means that makes language possible.

The forms of matter that inhabit a new integrative level, and the principles that characterize the functions of this matter usually evolve from a few forms and principles, chosen by natural selection, from the large variety of forms and principles available on the lower integrative level. Let us call this the *natural selection of forms,* and consider it a special case of the more general phenomenon of morphogenesis.

The manifestations of this policy along the physical interfaces are much less striking than they are along the higher ones, though examples can nevertheless be found. Leaving the eotemporal world for the biotemporal one, we note that the percentage composition by elements of living substance does not correspond either to that of the universe at large, or to that of the earth. Carbon, nitrogen, oxygen, hydrogen carry the great bulk of organic behavior, with a dozen or so other elements crucially but only minimally present. Going from life to man, we find that of the million and a half named species, and innumerable other species that died out, it is only a very few, perhaps only a single one that came to evolve the brain whose functions determine the nootemporal umwelt.

Let us mean by the "language" of an integrative level classes of signals and symbols in which the laws and regularities of nature must be expressed so as to satisfy the critical and practical intelligence of man, the formulator and tester of those laws. When so understood, we note *changes in language* as we cross the interfaces. In this view, languages are umwelt-specific, with each language incorporating those beneath it while adding some of its own peculiarities. Thus, the interfaces may be said to be semi-permeable to the languages of the integrative levels which they separate: information from below may be passed upward, but level-specific information from above cannot ordinarily penetrate to below. This is a non-reductionist stance, one that is essential to the theory of time as conflict, but it is a principle which cannot be rigorously proved; it can only be made increasingly plausible.

When the hierarchical asymmetry of languages is examined in detail, a good case can be made for distinguishing three different types of communications. Explanations given in a language appropriate for an umwelt can be usefully described as "intelligible" for the purposes of that umwelt. Signs and symbols appropriate to a higher umwelt may be described as "unintelligible" in terms of the lower language, while those appropriate for a lower integrative level are "obvious." For instance, the processes of natural selection working on the phenotype are intelligible in biotemporal language; the laws and regularities of molecules that make up the genes are intelligible in prototemporal and eotemporal language and obvious in biotemporal language. The symbolism of dreams is intelligible in nootemporal language but unintelligible in prototemporal language.

In the theory of time as conflict the unresolvability of certain conflicts, indigenous to an umwelt, are seen as the motive forces for the emergence of the next higher integrative level. The dynamics of this process may be discussed under the name of *conflicts and their resolutions*. When the specifics of the emergence of new umwelts are examined, it can be shown that it is along the interfaces (that is, among functions and structures that are metastable, that separate languages of integrative levels, etc.) where the complete failure, the fiasco of prior modes of conflict resolution become evident and the leading edge of the new integrative level is first manifest.

The essence of the physical conflicts may be implied by pointing to the opposition between the entropy increasing trends in inanimate nature expressed in the famous Second Law of Thermodynamics, and those specific laws of physics and chemistry which minimize that entropy increase. But, passive physical systems cannot be more efficient in opposing entropy increase than to make it minimal or even zero; in this condition I see the inadequacy of the physical mode of conflict resolution.

The limitation was overcome through the appearance of life, that is, through stable systems which decrease entropy locally. Life lasts only as long as the conflict lasts between the entropy increasing and decreasing trends; if and when this conflict vanishes living matter returns to its inanimate form. Conflict is thus seen to be immanent in life and unresolvable by means available within the biotemporal umwelt. Life itself ought then to be understood not as a one-way thrust of some kind but as a conflict between growth and decay.

But organic evolution is limited in the rate at which it can provide adaptation. In the plant world the rate of adaptation has been increasing throughout the evolution of the plant kingdom by such means, for instance, as the descendency of trees in general and the ascendency of shorter-lived plants; these latter can adapt most readily, hence faster, to available environmental niches. In the history of the evolution of the most advanced animal species the limitation of the rate at which evolutionary diversification can take place became a crucial issue, especially since the environment to which advanced life forms were to adapt became increasingly more complex because of the very success of organic evolution.

The limitations just implied were overcome through the capacity of the human mind to create symbolic transformations of experience. The mind can construct a symbolic continuity known as the "self." With the assistance of this symbol, and of all other symbols of our "inner landscape," it became possible to effect evolutionary changes without the need of going through the organic selection process.

However, the mind also has its own unresolvable conflicts: those between the expected and the encountered. A tension, or a difference between the expected and the encountered must be maintained if the identity of the self is to be retained. Should such conflict vanish for any length of time, the mind would begin to manufacture new goals and desires. If it is impossible to reestablish and maintain the conflict, the self collapses and nootemporality vanishes: a person becomes senile or insane. But the functioning of the individual mind leads to a dead end whenever its expectations get too far away from the conditions encountered. This conflict gives rise to yet a new integrative level, that of the sophisticated machinery of the societal umwelt.

3. FROM SMALL COLLECTIVES TO A GLOBAL SOCIETY

We have just identified certain systematic conditions associated with transitions between adjacent stable integrative levels: metastability, new uses for old functions and structures, natural selection among forms, changes in language and, finally, the resolution of lower order conflicts. I propose to use these policies as guidelines in discussing time's rite of passage from the temporalities of individuals and collectives of limited size to the temporality of a global collective of man. I shall deliberately neglect the tremendous multiplicity of social times that are normally discussed in time in sociology, for my interest is to find how all these temporalities, as a class, differ from the temporality of a possible worldwide community of man. We already know that the temporality of each stable level is rich: the time of an earthworm is quite distinct from that of a frog, which is distinct from that of a chimpanzee but, as a group, biotemporality is distinct from prototemporality, or eotemporality. It is in this, gross sense and without a fine structure that I seek the hallmarks of a transience of time from individual to the potential, common umwelt of all people on earth. The reasons for my limiting the use of "society" to a global collective relate to an observation, an opinion, and an assumption.

The observation is that the mutual interdependence among individuals and nations in the world community has been increasing at a rapid rate. This increase is encouraged by a call for a universal industrial civilization which, eventually, will not be able to function within areas smaller than the total surface of the earth. It would demand a multiple, communicative interconnectedness and organization that will surely cement its members into a functioning, single whole.

The opinion is that such a world society, if it should come about, would in fact constitute a new integrative level of nature. I have argued recently that when the brain, in its evolution, reached a certain degree of complexity it gave rise to the integrative level of the mind, which is capable of producing other minds of equal or superior sophistication via its network of signs and symbols. Likewise, I believe that when this network of signs and symbols reaches a certain complexity, we may look for the emergence of a new integrative level, the societal.

The assumption is that the interface between the individual mind (the noetic umwelt) and the societal umwelt would, in fact, follow the policies that the lower interfaces do.

I shall now take up the five policy features that we have just identified and make some guesses regarding their significance in the context of an emerging family of man.

(a) NEW USES FOR OLD FUNCTIONS

We are going to go back and forth between individual and societal functions.

During organic evolution the nervous system of man, including his brain, became so well adapted to its role as the coordinator of the functions of an individual that it has not yet stopped expanding its executive domain. It tends to extend the limits of its boundaries by coordinating groups of individuals into society. I believe that since the brain is already of such complexity as is possible to produce by biological means, what we have been doing during the evolution of historic man is learning how to put this complexity to better use. The societal extension of the functions of the mind is part of that learning process. By "mind" I understand the process description of the brain; "behavior" may then be interpreted as the acting out of certain brain states.

The internal happenings that correspond to behavior would be the signals carried in the brain by appropriate neural codes, with the brain itself the immediate environment of the mind. The most direct and richest representation of the internal codes of the brain is, surely, the spoken and written tongue: it enables the individual to formulate and establish his identity and tie this symbolic continuity to the symbolic continuities that we know as "other selves." This method of establishing identity is projected into the world of the collectives of man where it assists in the creation and perpetuation of that new symbolic continuity which we call mankind.

Just as the brain may be said to be the environment of the mind, so collectives of individual minds form the environment of the societal umwelt. It is individuals that generate, provide for the transmission, and exchange the signs and symbols appropriate to the new integrative level of society. The network of these symbols is the ancient and modern means of communication. By sound and light modulation, by electric and mechanical signals communication does for society what the neural network does for the individual. The use of societal symbols and signs in the establishment of the collective identity is then one example of a new use for already existing functions.

In the model of the mind which I developed some time ago, it was useful to postulate the workings of two imaginary actors: the Observer and the Agent. These two actors represented, respectively, the evolutionarily older, eotemporal function of the brain (that was the Observer) and its newer, nootemporal functions (that was the Agent). They were found to bear a hierarchical relation to one another and were said to be "distrustful" of each other's opinions. The tension and the communication between the two were found to display certain features which, taken together, suggested conscious experience and free will.

In the societal integrative level I discern a perennial struggle between the same two actors, in the ancient role of the "Prophet" and the "Statesman." The Prophet is rather like the Observer: he claims to be in command of knowledge concerning both future and past; hence surveys the affairs of man in terms of unchanging criteria. The Prophet's memories and expectations are certain and resemble the deterministic umwelt of eotemporality. The Statesman is rather like the Agent. His time is asymmetrical because his future contains certain irreducible uncertainties with which he must deal in a crucial present. Just as with the Agent and the Observer for the individual mind, so with Statesman and Prophet, it is their interaction, dialogues, enmities, trusts and mistrusts that set the fate of the societal body of which they are part; except that in the societal setting the two individuals need not be and usually are not the same person.

The separation of a single mind into two imaginary actors is, of course, an analytical trick; it is only the underlying existential tension that can be given ontic status. But that some of the functions of the indivdual mind, when projected across the interface break up into components which then materialize as two distinct persons, is an example of the evolutionary division of labor, a policy of evolution well known in the development of complex organisms.

There are many other examples for new uses of old functions and structures, carried across the interface between man and society by division of labor. Technology, for instance, is a communal enterprise that extends the bodily functions of man in certain ways that no individual, working alone, could possibly match. Science, as distinct from technology, is yet another example. It is a collective enterprise in search for knowledge which communal judgment may hold to be true, that is, unchanging through time. Science engages the capacities of the individual minds but directs them into domains which are unthinkable in a world of independent individual selves, no matter how ingenious each individual might be. Even ethics may be interpreted as a collective experimentation with the imagery of the individual mind, an enterprise which is quite meaningless except in a communal framework.

It seems, then, that political, scientific, and ethical practices, though originating in the mind of the individual, form a language which is that of the societal and not of the noetic integrative level.

(b) NATURAL SELECTION OF FORMS

Let us first consider some characteristics of the lower interfaces. For instance, the chemical composition of living matter is quite different from the natural abundance of elements of inanimate matter in the crust of the earth, even though life did arise from the earth; or, the human mind is quite uncharacteristic of living forms in general, even though man evolved from among all other living creatures. Out of what elements should we expect the leading forms of the societal integrative level to be selected? Out of symbolic continuities ordinarily referred to as "ideas?" I do not mean disembodied ghosts, but rather the actual world of signals that communicates ideas among men. They determine an umwelt as distinct from that of the individual mind, as the nootemporal umwelt of the mind is distinct from the biotemporal one of the brain.

Without detailed deliberation one cannot even guess which specific ideas might comprise the major form of the societal world, but it is possible to make two observations.

One concerns the symbolic continuity of the private self: that curious construct which is believed to operate in the world external to its body, yet without a completely identifiable external referent. Group identity is an analogous construct. It is defined and continuously refined by conflict, and by comparison with the collective identities of other groups. "One nation, indivisible, under God" is thinkable only in the company of other nations, equally indivisible. For the societal Umwelt, that is, for the family of man, this process of definition, by comparison, is not available, because there are no other humanities against which the identity of a global society could be defined. It is very likely, therefore, that the selection of the major forms which are to constitute the societal umwelt will run up against problems that have no parallel among the lower interfaces. This, I suppose, is one of the many great difficulties unique to the study of societal behavior.

The other observation is that in all lower umwelts, for the selection process to work, it was necessary to have a large store of different elements upon which to operate. Although only a relatively few forms were then carried on into the initial structures of the next higher integrative level, the continued existence of other elements remained a necessity. It may thus be speculatively inferred that if a societal umwelt were to emerge around a few central ideas, it will be able to retain viability only if it remains submerged in a sufficiently large store of ideas other than those upon which the identity of the family of man might be built. This is not so much an issue in sociology as it is in political science.

(c) CHANGE OF LANGUAGE

Methods of communication that are useful among individuals, such as the spoken, written and - in a more general sense - the acted-out languages, draw upon the biological and mental capacities of the individual; these are the languages appropriate for families, tribes and nations. Would the same languages be appropriate for the societal integrative level which I envision as arising from the noetic world? I do not believe so. But I am not thinking of such trivialities as, for instance, the diplomatic language used among heads of state, but rather of the fact that individuals prefer to communicate with individuals. Franz Kafka's K had great difficulties in crossing the communication boundaries between himself and the different language spoken by the Castle.

I characterized the asymmetry of languages about low interfaces as "obvious," when looking down, as "intelligible" when looking around, and as "unintelligible" or "mystical" when looking upward. Let us consider a few examples from the relationships between the individual and society.

Certainly, the replacement of individual values by collective values is often unintelligible. Again, I do not mean such easily identifiable practices as the willful beclouding of issues by certain governments. Rather, I am thinking of the replacement of individual reality by collective reality, such as in interpreting the actions of man as an historical beast. The story of man is filled with more examples of senseless horror than, prorated per capita, we would admit as likely.

Theories that propose to account for the bloody discontents of civilizations in terms of the drives and pains of the individual might well reach the sources of such discontents but, precisely because they consider the individual alone and not society as a whole, they cannot account for the qualitative change, something more than the simple amplification of individual behavior, displayed in the historic actions of the masses. One contention of my talk tonight is that the regularities of mass behavior are those of the societal and not of the noetic umwelt.

These and similar issues have been discussed in philosophy under the rubric of holism vs. individualism. In sociology, certain related matters are known under the heading of "unintended results." Rather crassly, this is the problem of the soldier looking at his comrades: "If neither you nor I really want to be here, and if the people across the trench do not want to be here either, then why are we here?" What we have learned so far suggests that the sources of unintelligibility, and of possible feelings of mysteriousness, are to be sought in the epistemological asymmetry of the languages that surround the noetic/societal interface. That is, explanations of the regularities indigenous to the societal umwelt cannot be given in a totally satisfactory way in languages appropriate only to the umwelt of the individual mind.[4]

Consider the unfolding affairs of the world and witness the growing multitudes of people, increasingly joined by certain proposed uniform solutions of their common needs. The impression is unavoidable that the messages that carry their ideas have some functions of their own and possess a degree of freedom over and above those of the individual mind. Here, I believe, is one of the interesting entries for inquiries into strategies for intervention into public policies.

The asymmetry of languages is encountered not only while looking up, but also when looking downward, and there are many examples of such "downward" looks. Claims for the inferiority and insignificance of the individual as compared with the collective self have probably been made ever since man appeared, but it is only with the explosive growth of communication and the beckoning development of a single human community that the awesome ramifications of this lop-sided relationship comes into full view. Surely, whatever is beneficial to a world-wide society does not necessarily benefit the individual and vice versa. This asymmetry has often been noted, bemoaned, or praised in languages appropriate for the individual, for it is to him that such comments have traditionally been addressed. It is quite conceivable, however, and specifically suggested by the theory of time as conflict that if, and as, the world enters the state I called the sociotemporal umwelt, languages in which the plight of the individual might be expressed will retain no more significance than the voice of a scrambled egg has for the hen that laid it. The family of man may have no language left in which to express emotions associated with death and birth, or to allow for - and therefore make thinkable - the traditional rites of passage. Social time would then become something resembling eotemporality rather than nootemporality.[5]

(d) METASTABILITY

Things and processes that constitute the interfaces might be described as "unpopular" in that they do not properly belong to any of the stable integrative levels. But as we rise along the hierarchy of umwelts, they become more evident. That is, although as a class they are all metastable, as the complexity of their neighboring umwelts increase so does the identifiability of metastable processes. I would like to discuss now some evidence that suggests that as a family of man we are entering a metastable integrative state. My examples are drawn from thoughts on ethics.

Throughout the known history of man, instructions for praiseworthy conduct seem to have been around, regardless of the size of groups. That such instructions were apparently always needed suggests that conflicts betweeen the interests of communities and those of individuals accompanied the social history of man. In the social life of animals we can also find rules but, as far as one can tell, collective demands either do not elicit conflicts within the individual, or if they do, the conflicts do not have the potentiality of becoming creative forces; altruism, a currently popular term, is not to be confused with compassion. A young dog might lick an ailing, old dog, but dogs have no policy on aging. The reason for this profound difference between animal and human communities is the absence in animals of individual selves which could find themselves opposed to the collective self. The interest of the group and the interest of the individual coincide: the struggle of the individual against the identity of the species is either nonexistent or insignificant. In stark contrast, one way to interpret the history of man is in terms of the perennial struggle between individual and communal destinies.

As in the matter of language asymmetry and of the natural selection of form, the issues of the individual/societal interface come into sharp focus only with the changes that prepare the possible emergence of a world community. In traditional societies it was ordinarily much easier to be a rugged individual living in the Norse woods, *or* an essentially nameless member of a human anthill (small or large), than to be both, simultaneously. It is not easy to give to the King what is the King's and to the individual what is the individual's, for they are often mutually exclusive. Much thought and energy has been expended in modern times in the socially advanced portions of the world toward the establishment of a working order where individual and collective interests may be harmoniously reconciled. In terms of our prior findings, such a reconciliation, if achieved, would imply conditions that might prevail within, rather than below or above the noetic/societal interface.

If the policies of lower order interfaces are useful guides, a balance between the individual and the societal selves, when assumed to apply to a world-wide society, is at best a precarious and metastable condition; the prognosis for the duration of this developmental state as a world-wide condition is one of radical brevity. As were the first living things which did not survive at all, and as is the buffer zone between body and mind that survived as our unconscious, the balanced condition that must characterize the nootemporal/sociotemporal interface may only be very short lived developmentally, even if its remnant would survive among the structures and functions of the new integrative level.

4. TRANSITION BETWEEN TWO TEMPORALITIES

It is appropriate now to return explicitly to questions of times's current rite of passage.

Consider first that because the language of the nootemporal umwelt subsumes all lower languages, we should be expected to be able to make authoritative statements about temporalities below the noetic. I believe that we can do so. Certainly, our formal sentences about the physical world carry great authority, even if it is impossible for us to experience atemporality, proto-, or eotemporality, other than in terms of moods. We can also explore biotemporality with confidence, though our understanding of the temporal world of organisms in not as well grounded as is our understanding of lower temporalities. In spite of the difficulties of regressive sharing, however, we can at least approach in our own experience the temporal umwelts of higher animals. But when it comes to nootemporality, our knowledge seems to be almost entirely that of feeling rather than understanding. A degree of unintelligibility has been one of the hallmarks of questions pertaining to "the time of man."

It is one thing to talk about the end of a particular physical process, or the end of the life of a flea, or a rabbit, or someone else: is quite another thing to contemplate the end in time of my own self. It is, again, one thing for me to talk about the beginning of a chemical change, or the birth of a child, and something quite different to contemplate the past that preceded my conscious experience. It is fascinating to reflect upon the time of the prototemporal, just barely distinguishable from the spatial; or upon the pure asymmetry of the eotemporal, or upon the aging of frogs, flowers and human males in general: but whence derives in my own mind that emphatically asymmetrical attitude toward post-mortem and prepartum existence?

There are also other issues. For instance, the atemporal is understandable. The probabilistic causation of the prototemporal, once understood as a primitive connectivity, can be accomodated in our scheme of thought. The deterministic causation of the eotemporal is convincing and convenient, as are the multiple and final causations of the biotemporal. Causation in human life is intuitively given, but it is immensely difficult to comprehend it discursively. But how can I accommodate that paradoxical feeling which informs me that some of my actions can be, and have been, freely taken in a world of processes that function according to law?

Consider next the thrust of man's history. The past could not honestly be called unintelligible, yet neither is it truly intelligible. As far back as one can see, our species has been driven by aspirations whose goals it cannot hope to reach, yet cannot accept as unreachable, such as ethical needs for justice and demands for consummate beauty. The hierarchical structure of the world contemplated in the theory of time as conflict, suggests that answers to questions such as these may be had only after they have been formulated in the language of the integrative level above that of the mind, that is, in the language of the sociotemporal umwelt. I am not imagining that citizens of a "brave new world" would be more perceptive than we are, or even better informed; the opposite is more likely to be the case. What I am saying is that in the language appropriate to the societal umwelt some aspects of such issues that pertain to birth and death control, to free will and destiny, to the role of the individual vs. the collective self, which now elude even the keenest of minds, may be so stated as to become answerable by the collective. Perhaps what I am saying is that social change will bring about a societal language in which questions of societal time may be stated and answered in ways acceptable to a global societal structure of man.

In a very disturbing way, since the features of new temporal umwelts arise from regions left unrecognized by the epistemology of a lower level, working within the confines of nootemporal language it is not even possible to delineate which portions of the issues fall into this category. That is, it is not possible to identify which of our unanswered questions may be answerable "from above," as it were, and which shall, or at least may, find satisfactory explication within the world of the individual mind.

Let us recall the unresolvable conflicts of the mind: those between the expected and the encountered, between passion and knowledge. Shakespeare put it this way in *Troilus and Cressida:*
...that the will is infinite, and the execution confined;
that the desire is boundless and the act slave to limit.

This conflict may be resolved by collapse: a man may become senile or lose his mind; the nootemporal then returns to the biotemporal. Or the conflict may be maintained. Doing so without self-destruction is usually regarded as a sign of the maturity of the ego. But, in our epoch something is happening in the nootemporal umwelt that resembles the condition of life's cul-de-sac which gave rise to the emergence of the mind. This time it is the individual mind which cannot function rapidly and efficiently enough; it cannot adapt to an environment which changes by the very deeds of the collectives of the individual minds. This, then, is the fiasco of the capacity of the individual self to deal with its own unresolvable conflict. The theory of time as conflict would identify such conditions as suggestive for the emergence of a new integrative level which, in some sense, would resolve the conflicts of the lower level.

There are many observations one can make that reinforce the suspicion that the family of man is indeed entering into a developmental state that belongs in the class of umwelts which I have described as interfaces.

Let the sensitivity of playwrights be our guide. The change in modern self is reflected, as one example, in the change of prevailing dramatic forms: in our epoch tragedy has come to be replaced by comedy, or, at best, by something of an "applied pathos," resembling uncomfortably closely the "passion surrogate" of the *Brave New World*.[6] In *Romeo and Juliet* society is reprimanded for its assumption of preeminence over the individual; whereas in the plays of Becket the individuals are punished for assuming preeminence over society.

During the period of history just preceding our epoch, much ingenuity was expended on devising means whereby the often opposing interests of the individual and of society might be reconciled. A foremost representative of these efforts is the American Constitution. The governmental structure that derived from the power of this document may be described as one whose primary task is to maintain a continuous reconciliation between individual and collective interests and among segments of government. By chance and historial good luck, and by the surviving genius of skillful compromise, the government so constituted succeeded in permitting and encouraging a condition of permanent revolution, one that was able to maintain and contain within boundaries the conflicts between the nootemporal and the sociotemporal worlds. But this mode of checks and balances is now under challenge from doctrines which define the individual entirely in terms of its position within the social collective.

The division of labor advocated by these doctrines demands the interchangability of people within occupations, thereby forcing the mind of man to operate in the world resembling the prototemporal umwelt of indistinguishable particles. Human anthills are in the making: some drab, some grey, some many-colored, but anthills just the same. Kafka's Castle is being exported from its natural habitat to the new and even newer world, distributed and promoted by the unholy alliance of opportunistic ideologies, international terrorism, and multinational corporations. As in the gastrulation of embryos, so also different groups of man are shifting around in search for, or anticipation of their final position, in the family of man. The traditional bonds of solidarity are dissolved under the pressure of industrial ethics which, ironically, has its sources in Christian soteriology, intended for the salvation of the individual. Some would say that such a new unity of mankind will surely be a nightmare, some perhaps that it will represent a Taoist seamless unity between the two cosmoses: that of society and that of the universe. My opinion is that in a global family of man there would be no personal identity left to which a harmony with nature might appear either as pleasing or repulsive.

"Now it is time that we were going," said Socrates, "I to die and you to live, but which of us has the happier prospect is unknown to anyone but God." The Socratic puzzle has not been answered but bypassed; its unresolvable conflict is on its way to resolution through the interchangability of individuals. It has been prophesied that there will be one fold and one shepherd, but the mental image that used to go with this prophecy has changed.

There are numerous manifestations of contemporary national and international life that suggest the transiency of our epoch. I mentioned some of them in passing, others I have discussed elsewhere.[7] Here I wish only to identify some by single sentences. They would surely sound strange to an Old Testament prophet praying for the unity of man one earth.

— Profound interference with the development of individual personalities through the direct modulation of sexual standards: the new sexual ethics.

— Radically increased fine structuring in the division of labor: Eve unbound.

— Human anthills in the making: interchangability of people within occupations.

—Impersonality of suffering and death: the replacement of the personal with a statistical Christ.

—Camera replacing pen, voice replacing printing: the media revolution.

—Silencing the classic struggle between statesman and prophet.

—Questioning the principle of checks and balances: the American experiment.

—Questioning the relevance of the past: world without history.

—Explosive increase of "mind-made" (artificial, invented) surrogates: applied pathos instead of tragedy, machine made music.

—Economic oscillations related to the uniqueness of global society: no other humanity against which the global identity of man may be defined.

The theory of time as conflict can say nothing about the actual future development of the relationship between individual and society. One can only guess what societal policy might teach about beginnings and endings (that is, births and deaths) for the citizens of the world; or what the detailed implementations might be for our attitudes toward aging and suffering, or even toward the social process itself. But it does seem to me that time's rite of passage from individual to society is a suitable focus for social scientific research and theory.

We may take courage and assert, however, that the type of balance in which we find ourselves today is metastable. Accordingly, the theory suggests two possible paths, based on what we have learned about lower order interfaces. The unresolvable conflicts of the mind may be resolved by the emergence of a new integrative level, that of the societal umwelt; or else, resolved by regression to the noetic umwelt of the individual minds grouped in tribes and families; or else, even by regression to the biotemporal, leaving the earth for the beasts that crawl, fly and swim.

What I have described as the metastability of the noetic/societal interface is not to be identified with any of the classical ideas of revolution. For it is not the revolt of the hungry against the well fed, or that of one race against another or one nation against another, and not even one ideology against another, although it includes all of these. Rather, it is a revolt against the unresolvable conflicts of the mind.

Hence, the march is not to the tune of Dies Irae, or to the Marseillaise, not even to that of the Communist Internationale, but to something much more elemental. We are in a metamorphosis wherein, as Kazantzakis put it "life has grown more savage, and the gods grown more powerful."

NOTES AND REFERENCES

1. J. T. Fraser, *Time as Conflict; a Scientific and Humanistic Study* (Basel: Birkhauser, 1978). See its references for prior history and elaboration of the idea.
2. The extended umwelt principle helps us get around the following thorny issue. In social process the individual is both an observer and a participant and therefore, one may argue, his reliability can be quesitoned. Consider, however, that this is but one example of the broad issue of knower and the known. We are made up of the same matter whose properies we seek in chemistry and physics, and we possess minds whose functions we seek to understand in psychology. The extended umwelt principle identifies ontology with the carefully examined limits of different epistemological domains and thus admits our intrinsic limitations - and takes it from there.
3. Including the evolution of machinery to manufacture complex molecules which cannot be found in non-living matter.
4. Here the stance of the theory of time as conflict is one opposing methodological individualism and maintaining the irreducibility of certain societal concepts, while also giving reasons why is it difficult to tell which concepts are truly irreducible and which ones are irreducible only because of our ignorance. Thus it is in agreement with much of the reasoning offered by Maurice Mandelbaum in "Societal Facts" and Steven Lukes in "Methodological Individualism Reconsidered," both in Slan Ryan, *ed., The Philosophy of Social Explanation* (Oxford: the University Press, 1973). This footnote was inserted following Professor Glassner's question (see *Discussion*). I am grateful for his comments and feel like the proverbial man who finally discovered that through all his life he has been speaking in prose.
5. Professor Barry Schwartz offered an anecdotal example to illustrate this point. (Personal communication). After the tragic death of the daughter of a friend, the colleagues of the bereaved father took extra-ordinary trouble to avoid him. Many interpretations are possible to account for this disturbing shyness, and possibly many are simultaneously true. The one favored by the

man himself was that the avoidance was an expression of sympathy in a society that does not provide its members with a vocabulary of condolence.
6. Cf. Gregor Sebba "Time and the modern self: Descartes, Rousseau, Beckett" and Tamas Ungvari "Time and the modern self: a change in dramatic form." Both in *The Study of Time I,* J.T. Fraser, F.C. Haber and G.H. Müller, *eds.* (Berling, Heidelberg, New York: Springer Verlag, 1972).
7. Fraser, *op. cit.* 263-80.

K. MARSHALL: I noticed similarities between what you are saying and many very esteemed philosophers, but in particular I noticed a parallel to ideas of Teilhard de Chardin in *The Phenomenon of Man.*

FRASER: There are similarities between the theory of time as conflict and Teilhard's evolutionism, just as there are similarities between that theory and Hegelian or Marxist dialectic. But the differences are fundamental. Teilhard sees what he calls "noosphere," a thinking layer on earth, which distinguishes man from the biosphere of other living things. There are certain parallels here. The idea itself is not really that new. But Teilhard perceives in the emergence of a hypersonal consciousness the final, terminal, Omega point of evolution which may or may not be identical with God, in his theory. Time as conflict sees the world as open-ended and evolution in terms of certain principles which permit such an open-ended evolution with no necessary uppermost level. And as far as the similarity and dissimilarity to Hegelian-Marxist dialectic is concerned, it is this. The theory does not see in the world a series of theses and anti-theses and syntheses but rather universal process which is somewhat isomorphic with advanced forms of reproduction: the unresolvable conflicts are coemergent with the unpredictably new.

K. MARSHALL: The particular aspect of de Chardin's conscious level was his view of increasing complexity and consciousness and your theory seemed to me to be increasing awareness of increasing complexity of time.

FRASER: Increasing complexity yes, increasing consciousness of time, no. When one holds that there may exist an increasing consciousness of time, the model of time one is forced to use is

Newtonian: a pre-existing time which flows without regard to events or things, and of which it is possible to become increasingly aware. In a theory of time as conflict there is no such a priori time. Instead, time itself is seen to evolve from the atemporal to the proto-, eo-, bio-, noo and sociotemporal, and perhaps beyond. This appears self-contradictory. But its logical consistency is guaranteed by the extended umwelt principle. That principle identifies the ways in which the world appears to us through the various ways of knowing, with the world as it is. It identifies the epistemic with the ontic. All this involves many other matters, let us say, operational issues, such as the difficulty of regressive sharing. We can understand the lower temporalities but it is difficult to experience them, to feel them. There are good reasons for this. They reside in the profound problems we would have if we could easily share these temporalities, experientially. But they may be expressed through certain moods, such as in the arts and letters.

GLASSNER: Concerning the sharing of lower temporalities, am I understanding correctly, that you claim we can better understand the lower temporalities?

FRASER: I think this is what happens. The lower temporalities we appreciate through understanding: those of radio waves, and of particles, of massive matter etc. As we rise to the temporalities of life in its increasingly complexifying forms, we are able to share, or feel what we are talking about better and better. The hope an animal seems to express through behavior is something we can feel ourselves. When it comes to the time of man, nootemporality, it is almost entirely feeling and very little understanding. If we look at this progression as reflecting our own status along the evolutionary ladder, then we have a diachronic system. This diachronic spectrum has its synchronic equivalent. I called it the Augustinian Uncertainty Principle. Paraphrased: "if you ask me what time is, I do not know; if you don't ask me, I do know," that is, I do feel. At one extreme of the spectrum we think, as in mathematical physics, and we have beautiful statements about formal time but the experience of time is all gone out of it. At the other end of the spectrum we have the totally experiential time of continuous becoming, of ecstasy. What is time in ecstasy? The answer is usually "I just can't tell you." So we have the two extremes: time understood and time felt; knowledge and passion. In daily life we try to strike a balance between the two extremes.

GLASSNER: Is it not that we are better capable of understanding the lower level because, after all, we invent the language we use to understand it. Language is simplification. So is it not that we are willing to "oversimplify" those levels? And if that is the case, is it not also the case that the linearity of your theory would be put in question?

FRASER: I don't think we have here a simplification by design or ignorance. Rather, it is a fact that the world itself is simpler as we approach the lower integrative levels. Again, this goes back to identifying the epistemic with the ontic. If the world of indistinguishable particles appears probabilistic, and it remains so after diligent search (and I can't put a definition on what is "diligent" or "sufficient" enough), then that part is implicit in the Copenhagen interpretation of quantum theory. I have extended that type of interpretation to other levels of nature. So we have the atemporality, prototemporality etc. Now, I derive a degree of encouragement from the further fact that an identical hierarchy of temporalities may be identified in the topology of the microstructure of time perception, in the development of the sense of time in the child, and even in the history of ideas.

V. MARSHALL: I think this relates to what you just said. To what extent do you rely upon anology for your argument, as opposed to relying on evidence. It seems to me that a great deal of your vision of the future rests on an extension of principles from lower orders, and I find your argument unconvincing in terms of evidence.

FRASER: When it comes to speculating about the future, as I have done, I know of no method whereby I could produce evidence. I can only say what I think might happen and give my reasons. One can then argue about the reasons, or even point to the fact that in cases of uncertainty people speculate in ways consistent with their temperaments, their world-views. Yes, I do work with analogy and with induction, and both so selected that they are in harmony with my temperament, training, etc.

V. MARSHALL: What I'm wondering is, why do you envision the emergence of a kind of societal world level that seems highly integrated, with a high degree of intercommunication holding it together? I wonder if perhaps the historical evidence argues against this. I may be swayed by the fact that I'm a Canadian. We're having enough trouble in our own society. I think of Wilber--the world is a social system--and I weigh that against the current of nationalism and so forth. These examples are at a much more concrete level than what you argue.

FRASER: Opinions about the future must, of course, depend on the data one selects as relevant and that, to an extent, as I just said, is a matter of world-views. But given the extreme difficulty of the issues, I was as concrete as it was possible to be. I did not try to predict which way the world will in fact go. Rather, from general policies established through a systematic review of what we do know about the emergence of new integrative levels, I said that the world is likely to go one of two ways, and is most unlikely to remain in a transient, metastable state. There are the centrifugal forces of a global society, such as the demand for Irish Power, Canadian French Power, Canadian Scottish Power etc. etc., a general trend of fragmentation. Simultaneously, there is a demand for world-wide uniformity because of the needs of goods etc. which pushes us in the direction of a global unity of man. I speculated that as the intensity of these two opposing trends increases, the world situation will become less and less stable.

HALL: I have two unrelated questions. First, is there a history at the level of particle matter, and if not, why not?

FRASER: To me "history" is primarily that of man but I believe you mean the reconstructed past of men, lions, frogs, moons, clouds, electrons etc. If history is understood as the possibility of this reconstruction of the past, in the series past-present-future, then, if you remain within the atemporal, prototemporal, eotemporal worlds, then history cannot exist. I can reconstruct and assign a history to the moon but if I imagine a world with moons and particles and light only, in that world "history" cannot be given any meaning. For instance, physics is totally ahistorical in two senses. The one, which is not the one we are now talking about, resides in the fact that the history of physics is irrelevant to present work, or almost so. That is not the point. Physics is ahistorical in the more important sense that the equations of physics, the physicist's t, does not allow for a present, a future, or a past.

HALL: Is that on a theoretical level or on a level of facts?

FRASER: Theory and fact amount to the same thing. Kepler's theory of planetary motion, embodied in his famous equations, cannot allow for history. Hence it is regarded to be a fact that planteray motion cannot have a history - from within physics.

HALL: The second question has to do with your positing of a societal umwelt as imaginary, and I'm wondering whether you're not skipping an actualized or a number of actualized quasisocietal levels, that is, levels of social groupings?

FRASER: Yes. My approach in this paper is definitely schematic. Each stable integrative level has, let's call it, a "fine structure." And this structuring itself becomes rapidly richer as we advance along the evolutionary ladder. The temporal umwelt of a tick is quite poor compared with, and certainly quite different from, that of a seeing eye dog, or an advanced ape. Ticks, seeing-eye dogs, grasshoppers, jackdaws were VexKull's favorite examples. So that is within the integrative level of life. Then on to mind: the temporal umwelts of individuals have much in common, that's why it can be described by one name, but in some ways there must be as many kinds as there are individuals. To society, yes, perhaps every tribe, nation, ethnic group has something peculiar to its societal umwelt.

SCHWARTZ: As I understand it, you are arguing that each level of integration of matter has certain temporal characteristics. For example, the temporal properties of the human brain, described as the most complex structure in the universe. You record the mind as being a process-description of the brain. Now these temporal properties include the conflict between the expected and the encountered. They include expectation, memory, dread and so forth. I also take it that the sociotemporal level has its own properties. What are these properties? And how do these properties differ from the temporal properties of the mind?

FRASER: I cannot list such properties, I do not know them. But I have some suggestions as to which direction to look: socially acceptable answers to birth and death control that is, beginnings and endings. They are strictly temporal issues. Attitudes toward the individual vs. society. Attitudes toward the traditional rites of passage. If the rites of adolescence, or marriage, or baptism, or death are eliminated - how can time be conceptualized by the individual? Also, about this matter of just what sociotemporality will comprise, there is a clear epistemological issue and I mentioned that in the paper. I believe that it is difficult, if not impossible, to describe in the language of an integrative level some of the features of a higher integrative level. So first I would look to the emergence of a language that is appropriate for the family of man. Then certain issues of sociotemporality will become discussable in that language.

DAVIS: You, of course, have had to compress very much into one short lecture and I cannot say that I understand what strikes me as an obviously exciting natural philosophy of evolution, and perhaps some of my comments reflect on my misunderstanding. I suspect that one of the implications that the sociologist or social historian would take from your theory, if it were accepted, is that we could look at history in an evolutionary perspective. What I would like to suggest is that I don't think that's a useful perspective for a sociologist or anyone who wants to look at the behavior of men. It is a perspective which, unfortunately, has reduced much of sociology. The evolutionary perspective that I think your theory implies for sociologists entails some kind of cumulative effect that is orderly. Of course, the present in some way is built upon the past, but not in a lawful way, and while you say that history is open-ended, I could agree with that, too, in the sense that it is random. I'll give you one real example, the history of torture. In the 13th and 14th centuries in Great Britain, torture was explicitly outlawed by the common law of Great Britain. By the Tudor monarchy it was introduced lawfully--and it was the famous introduction of the rack. Now if we would take the normal kind of stereotypic view of human behavior, we call torture uncivilized and the prohibition against torture as civilized, here we have a society mov-

ing from a level of civilization to a level of lesser civilization. So
I would like to see how you can take those events and put them
in an evolutionary perspective?

FRASER: You are familiar with Bronowski's popular idea of
an "ascent of man." He identified man's history with the history
of technology and since technical and scientific knowledge are
cumulative, so, in his view, is the ascent of man. He mistakes
the history of science for the history of man. Banish the
thought! I don't want to be in the same boat. But I do insist that
during the last fifteen million years, or whatever, our particular
species has learned how to use his brain, and thus an evolutionary view, if it is not taken to mean a pre-determined path to
Teilhard's Omega point, certainly makes sense. The issue is too
complex to be dealt with in the form of questions and answers;
let's talk about it separately.

GLASSNER: I'd like to pick up on one part of Professor Davis'
questions and take it in a slightly different direction: that's the
problem of methodological individualism, or the idea that in
order to know society, you must derive that knowledge from
understanding the individual. It strikes me that you have a subtle form of methodological individualism when you derive your
theory by taking the functions that you find in the lower and
then saying that they become transformed into the higher.

FRASER: I fear I do not know what is meant by "methodological individualism" so I cannot comment on it, but I will try to
find it out. (*Editor's note*: see Footnote 4 of the paper). I do not
know where this would fit in with "methodological individualism," but here is one thought. Personal identity is a symbolic structure. We handle the self as though it were altogether
in a world external to us, like other identities. "I am in the room
with tables and chairs and other people." But in fact it is partly
inside me and partly outside; I cannot explore myself as I can
explore other identities. Isomorphic arguments hold for society.
Any group for that matter - all butchers, all bakers, all candle-
stick makers - forms a symbolic continuity, as do nations and
even humanity at large. So there are some similarities between
the individual and society.

INDEX